CONCEPT MAPPING

A Critical-Thinking Approach to Care Planning

SECOND EDITION

Pamela McHugh Schuster, RN, PhD
Professor of Nursing
Youngstown State University
Youngstown, Ohio

 F. A. DAVIS COMPANY • Philadelphia

F. A. Davis Company
1915 Arch Street
Philadelphia, PA 19103
www.fadavis.com

Copyright © 2008 by F. A. Davis Company

Printed in the United States of America

Last digit indicates print number: 10 9 8 7 6 5 4 3 2

Publisher, Nursing: Joanne Patzek DaCunha, RN, MSN
Content Development Manager: Darlene D. Pedersen, MSN, APRN-BC
Senior Project Editor: Danielle J. Barsky
Cover Designer: Carolyn O'Brien

As new scientific information becomes available through basic and clinical research, recommended treatments and drug therapies undergo changes. The author(s) and publisher have done everything possible to make this book accurate, up to date, and in accord with accepted standards at the time of publication. The author(s), editors, and publisher are not responsible for errors or omissions or for consequences from application of the book, and make no warranty, expressed or implied, in regard to the contents of the book. Any practice described in this book should be applied by the reader in accordance with professional standards of care used in regard to the unique circumstances that may apply in each situation. The reader is advised always to check product information (package inserts) for changes and new information regarding dose and contraindications before administering any drug. Caution is especially urged when using new or infrequently ordered drugs.

Library of Congress Cataloging-in-Publication Data

Schuster, Pamela McHugh, 1953-
  Concept mapping : a critical-thinking approach to care planning /
Pamela McHugh Schuster. — 2nd ed.
       p.   ;   cm.
  Includes bibliographical references and index.
  ISBN 978-0-8036-1567-0 (alk. paper)
  1. Nursing. 2.   Critical thinking.   I. Title.
  [DNLM: 1.   Patient Care Planning. 2.   Audiovisual Aids. 3.   Concept Formation.
4.   Nursing Process—organization & administration.   WY 100 S395c 2008]
  RT42.S38 2008
  362.17'3068—dc22   2007017274

*This book is dedicated to nursing students
learning to organize patient-care planning
and to provide effective nursing care
as well as to the nursing students' clinical faculty.*

*The book is also dedicated to my husband, **Fred**,
and to my children, **Luke, Leeanna, Patty, Isaac,** and **Brent.***

CONCEPT MAPPING

A Critical-Thinking Approach to Care Planning

A NOTE ABOUT USAGE

To avoid both sexism and the constant repetition of "he or she," "his or her," and so forth, masculine and feminine pronouns are used alternately throughout the text.

PREFACE

Concept mapping is a diagrammatic teaching and learning strategy that allows students and faculty to visualize interrelationships among medical diagnoses, nursing diagnoses, assessment data, and treatments. Although concept mapping can be done in nursing lecture classes and can be used for diagramming diverse concepts in nursing and other disciplines, the purpose of this book is to use concept mapping theory to develop a patient care map as a guide for nursing care in clinical settings.

The concept care map comprises a five-step process. Before developing a care map, the student must perform a patient assessment. From the assessment data, the student develops a skeleton diagram of the patient's health problems (step 1). The student then analyzes and categorizes specific patient assessment data (step 2) and indicates relationships between nursing and medical diagnoses (step 3). In step 4, the student develops patient goals, outcomes, and nursing interventions for each nursing diagnosis. Step 5 is to evaluate the actual patient response to each nursing intervention and to summarize clinical impressions. Care mapping enables the student to recognize the relationships between medical and nursing care problems, including integration of pathology, medications, treatments, and laboratory and diagnostic testing. Using this care map process, the student:

▶ Identifies the primary patient care problems using specific evidenced-based assessments
▶ Analyzes patient profile data, categorizes data to describe problems, and documents each problem within a box on the care map
▶ Draws lines between boxes to indicate relationships
▶ Assigns numbers to the problems to indicate their priority
▶ Develops a goal, outcomes, and interventions for each problem
▶ Uses maps in the clinical setting to select appropriate interventions to provide effective care
▶ Writes notes on the maps to indicate evaluation of outcomes and keeps the maps current during the clinical day
▶ Uses clinical care maps as the basis for documentation in patient medical records

After the theoretical discussion of each step in developing the care map, the book presents scenarios and exercises that the student can use to practice the steps to gradually develop the ability to reason clinically and formulate accurate and complete nursing diagnoses and develop individualized plans of care. Because this process will be taught to students with varying amounts of clinical experience, the scenarios presented are not complex and cover common reasons for admission to hospital settings.

This Second Edition of *Concept Mapping* has been updated and revised based on my continued use of concept care maps in clinical settings and the recommendations of faculty and students who have been working with concept care maps since the First Edition. I wish you all much success in planning and implementing nursing care using this exciting new method of concept care maps to provide outstanding patient care.

REVIEWERS

Hobie Etta Feagai, MSN, APRN-BC, FNP
Assistant Professor
Hawaii Pacific University
Kaneohe, Hawaii

Bette M. Ferree, RN, MSN, ARRN-BC
Assistant Professor
Winston-Salem State University
Winston-Salem, North Carolina

Elaine Bishop Kennedy, EdD, RN
Professor
Wor-Wic Community College
Salisbury, Maryland

Mark Longshore, MSN, RN, FNP
Nursing Faculty
Front Range Community College
Ft. Collins, Colorado

Barbara Maxwell, MSN, MS, CNS, RN
Associate Professor of Nursing/Program
  Coordinator
SUNY Ulster
Stone Ridge, New York

Deena Nardi, PhD, APRN-BC, FAAN
Professor
Lewis University
Romeoville, Illinois

Victoria Queen, MSN, RN
Nursing Instructor
Greenville Technical College
Greenville, South Carolina

Joyce P. Shutt, RN, BS, MS
Nursing Instructor
Greenville Technical College
Greenville, South Carolina

Beverly Smith, RN, BSN
Faculty Vocational Nursing Program
San Jacinto College North
Houston, Texas

Barbara Tacinelli, MA, RN
Professor of Nursing
Borough of Manhattan Community
  College
New York, New York

Sharon Wahl, RN, BSN, MSNEd, EdD
Professor Emeritus
San Jose State University
San Jose, California

Jack Yensen, RN, PhD
Editor-in-Charge, *eLearning*
Online Journal of Nursing Informatics
Langara College
Victoria, British Columbia

CONTENTS

1

'TWAS THE NIGHT BEFORE CLINICAL...

OBJECTIVES

1. Define concept care maps.

2. List the purposes of concept care maps.

3. Identify the theoretical basis for concept care maps.

4. Relate critical thinking processes to the nursing process and to concept care maps.

5. Identify steps to develop a concept care map.

6. Describe how concept care mapping corresponds to the nursing process.

7. Identify how concept care maps are used during patient care.

8. Describe the purpose of standards of care as related to concept care maps.

9. List health-care providers and agencies responsible for developing and enforcing standards of care.

10. Describe the purpose of managed care.

'Twas the night before clinical, and all through the house, not a creature was stirring...except for you! There you are with books piled high around you trying to get ready to give safe and competent nursing care to the patients you have been assigned for the next morning. It is late, and you are tired. What if there was a way for all the information you have gathered on your patients to just "come together," make perfect sense, and form a simple, complete care plan? If you have ever found yourself in this situation, this book is for you. It was written to help you organize and analyze patient data quickly and efficiently and to develop a working care plan that is referred to as a concept *care* map. A concept care map is the plan used to give daily nursing care to a patient. Note the emphasis on the word *care*. The purpose of the map is to provide patient care. The concept care maps you develop for your patients will be practical and realistic; they will be implemented and evaluated during the clinical day. Best of all, there is very little writing to do. No more tedious writing of nursing care plans.

The purpose of this book is to teach you how to develop a concept care map, which is to be carried in your pocket on the clinical area and used in the care for your patient. In addition, it is very important to for you to understand how your performance and your concept care map will be evaluated by your clinical faculty.

The purpose of this chapter is to describe the theoretical basis for concept care maps and to provide an overview of what they are, how they are developed, and how they are used during patient care. In addition, the chapter introduces general standards for guiding and evaluating patient care within managed care systems. Managed care principles are used in almost all health-care delivery systems. The purpose of managed care is to decrease costs while maintaining the quality of health services. The implications of managed care are far-reaching, and they guide the development of nursing care plans. Later chapters will lead you step by step through each aspect of developing and using concept care maps.

What Are Concept Care Maps?

Concept care mapping is an innovative approach to planning and organizing nursing care. In essence, a concept care map is a diagram of patient problems and interventions. Your ideas about patient problems and treatments are the "concepts" that you will diagram. In this book, the term *concept* means idea. Developing clinical concept care maps will enhance your critical thinking skills and clinical reasoning because you will visualize priorities and identify relationships in clinical patient data clearly and succinctly. Concept care maps are used to:

▶ Organize patient data
▶ Analyze relationships in the data
▶ Establish priorities
▶ Build on previous knowledge
▶ Identify what you do not understand

▶ Enable you to take a holistic view of the patient's situation[1]

The templates for the concept care map are shown in Figures 1.1, 1.2, and 1.3. Take a few minutes to study them. You will be using these templates to outline patient problems; organize patient data on pathology, treatments, medication, laboratory data, and the patient's emotional state; develop goals and outcomes; and list what you will be doing to address each problem. Figure 1.1 is the "sloppy copy." You will be writing down short notations about a patient's problems by grouping data under problem areas. It does not have to be perfect. It takes time to think critically about how to categorize data correctly under problems, and sometimes you may change your mind about where data fit into the clinical picture you hare developing about your patient. The "final edition" in Figure 1.2 is the care plan you submit after the clinical day is over, after you have had more time to evaluate critically what happened during your clinical experiences with the patient. Bring your sloppy copy along with goals, outcomes, and interventions in Figure 1.3 to the clinical agency.

The Theoretical Basis of Care Mapping

Concept care maps have roots in the fields of education and psychology.[2,3] Concept maps have also been called cognitive maps, mind maps, and meta-cognitive tools for teaching and learning.[4,5] They have been used in many classroom settings as teaching tools to get important ideas to stick in the minds of students. Nursing educators have recognized the usefulness of this teaching/learning strategy in summarizing and visualizing important concepts, and there is a growing body of knowledge on this topic.[6-10]

From the field of education, Novak and Gowin[11] developed the theory of meaningful learning and have written about "learning how to learn." They have defined concept maps theoretically as "schematic devices for representing a set of concept meanings embedded in a framework of propositions." They further explain concept maps as hierarchical graphical organizers that serve to demonstrate the understanding of rela-

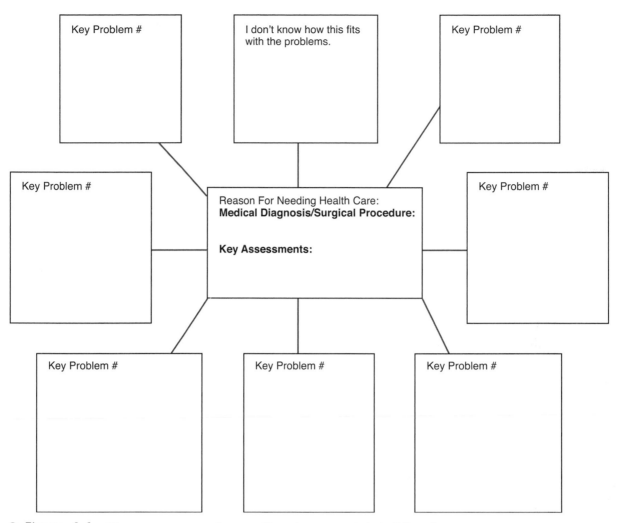

● Figure 1.1   Sloppy copy pre-conference. Carry in your pocket at all times!

tionships among concepts. This theoretical definition and explanation is highly abstract. Simply stated, concept maps are diagrams of important ideas that are linked together. The important ideas you need to link are patient problems and the pathophysiology, medications, laboratory data, and treatments for those problems. The concept maps you will be developing are for patients in clinical settings, so they are named concept care maps. You will use this special concept care map to guide the care of patients.

The educational psychologist Ausubel[12] has also contributed to the theoretical basis of concept mapping through the development of assimilation theory. Concept maps help those who write them to assimilate knowledge. The premise of this theory is that new knowledge is built on preexisting knowledge, and new concepts are integrated by identifying relationships with those concepts already understood. Simply stated, we build and integrate new knowledge into what we already know. By diagramming, you build the structure about the relationships in a concept. Concept maps help to identify and integrate what you already know. In addition, they can help reveal what you do not know or understand. This means that although you have ideas about patient problems or treatments, you may not be sure how those problems and treatments should be integrated into a comprehensive plan. Once you recognize what you do not understand and can formulate questions, you can seek out informa-

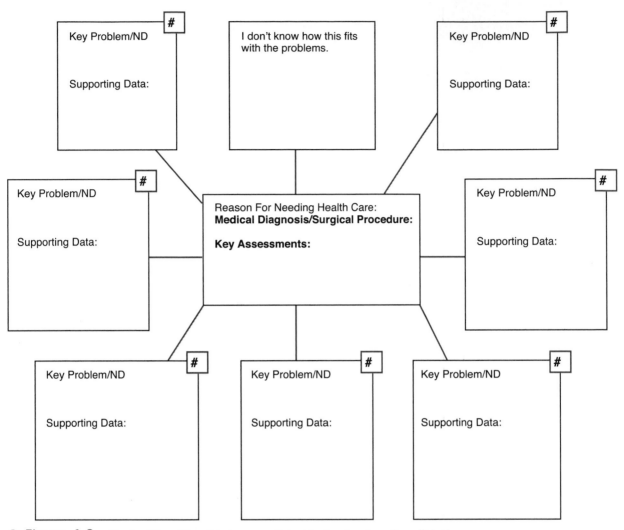

● Figure 1.2   Final edition. Give this to your clinical instructor day after clinical.

tion. Concept care maps help identify what you know and what you need to learn to provide quality patient care. The concept care map you create will evolve as you continue to assess and intervene with your patient. You will be adding to the concept care map throughout the clinical day.

Concept Care Mapping and Critical Thinking Yield Clinical Planning

Concept care mapping requires critical thinking. A widely accepted view of critical thinking by many nurse educators was developed by the American Philosophical Association: "Critical thinking is the process of purposeful, self-regulatory judgment. This process gives reasoned consideration to evidence, contexts, con-

ceptualization, methods, and criteria."[13] In developing a clinical concept care map, critical thinking is used to analyze relationships in clinical data. Thus, critical thinking used in developing concept care maps builds clinical reasoning skills. Critical thinking and clinical reasoning are used to formulate clinical judgments and decisions about nursing care. In 2000, the National League for Nursing Accrediting Commission's Report on Planning for Ongoing Systematic Evaluation and Assessment of Outcomes defined critical thinking specific to the discipline of nursing as "The deliberative *non-linear* process of collecting, interpreting, analyzing, drawing conclusions about, presenting, and evaluating information that is both factually and belief based."[14] Concept care maps are nonlinear and are used to

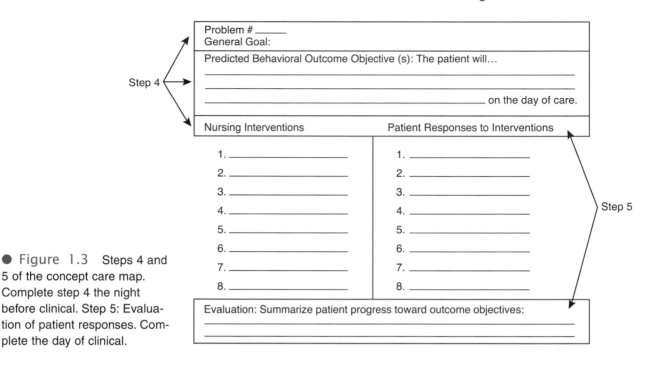

Problem # _____
General Goal:

Predicted Behavioral Outcome Objective (s): The patient will…
_____
_____
_____ on the day of care.

Nursing Interventions	Patient Responses to Interventions
1. _____	1. _____
2. _____	2. _____
3. _____	3. _____
4. _____	4. _____
5. _____	5. _____
6. _____	6. _____
7. _____	7. _____
8. _____	8. _____

Step 4

Step 5

Evaluation: Summarize patient progress toward outcome objectives:
_____
_____

● Figure 1.3   Steps 4 and 5 of the concept care map. Complete step 4 the night before clinical. Step 5: Evaluation of patient responses. Complete the day of clinical.

collect, interpret, analyze, present, and evaluate patient information.

Although concept maps have been used in a number of different ways in various disciplines, the focus of this book is on developing concept care maps for the purposes of clinical nursing care planning. You need to organize the concept care map prior to the care of the patient, which will help you organize and prioritize what needs to be done to promote optimal patient outcomes for the clinical day of care. The important ideas that must be linked together are the medical and nursing diagnoses, along with all pertinent clinical data, including the subjective and objective physical and emotional problems and underlying pathology, medications, laboratory data, and treatments. Concept care maps can be used to promote critical thinking and clinical reasoning about patient problems and treatment of problems. Through concept care mapping of diagnoses and clinical data, you can evaluate what you know about the care of a patient and what further information you need to provide safe and effective nursing care.[15]

Take, for instance, a situation where a certain drug or treatment does not make any sense to you as you analyze the entire clinical picture. It is very important to ask questions to your clinical faculty about what does not seem to fit the clinical picture, because the questions you ask can result in avoiding medication or treatment errors. In the past, there have been times when patients needed changes in the medications or treatments based on the findings of nursing students. So never hesitate to ask questions of your faculty. It is so important, in fact, that a special place has been provided on the care map template labeled "I don't know how this fits with the clinical problems." Place any information that you do not understand in this box. Perhaps there are drugs you cannot find in your references the night before clinical, or you may wonder why a patient needs a particular drug or treatment. The visual concept care map diagram of relationships among diagnoses allows you and your clinical faculty to exchange views on why relationships exist among problems and the treatments. It also allows you and your faculty to recognize the need for further assessment and questioning to avoid medication or treatment errors.

Overview of Steps in Concept Care Mapping

The nursing process is the foundation of the concept care map or any other type of nursing care plan. The nursing process involves assessing, diagnosing, planning, implementing, and evaluating nursing care. These steps are related to the development of concept care maps and the use of care plans during patient care in clinical settings. Subsequent chapters will give the details of care mapping with learning activities; this chapter presents an initial overview.

Preparation for Concept Care Mapping

Before developing a concept care map, the first thing you must do is gather clinical data. This step corresponds to the assessment phase of the nursing process. You must review patient records to determine current health problems, medical histories, physical assessment data, medications, and treatments. This assessment must be complete and accurate because it forms the basis for the concept care map. You may have the opportunity to meet a patient briefly the night before you begin care. In just 5 minutes of interacting with a patient—even by simply introducing yourself and watching the patient's response—you can gain a wealth of information about the patient's mood, level of comfort, and ability to communicate. Chapter 2 will focus on how to gather this clinical data.

Step 1: Develop a Basic Skeleton Diagram

Based on the clinical data you collect, you begin a care map by developing a basic skeleton diagram of the reasons your patient needs health care. The initial diagram is composed of clinical impressions you make after reviewing all the data. Write the patient's reason for seeking care (usually a medical diagnosis in a hospital setting) in the middle of the template in Figure 1.4. Then, around this central diagnosis, arrange the problems that you have determined based on your assessments—these represent the patient's responses to the patient's specific reasons for seeking health care. The final version of this template can be seen in Figure 1.5. The general problem statements will eventually be written as nursing diagnoses as shown in Figure 1.6.

The American Nurses Association (ANA) Social Policy Statement[16] indicates that the focus of nursing practice is on human responses to health states. The concept care map diagram reflects the ANA practice policy statement because the human responses are located around the health state of the patient. Nursing care will be focused on the human responses.

The central figure of the concept care map diagram contains the reason the patient is seeking health care—the reason for the hospitalization, extended care, or visit to the outpatient center. In this example, the health problem for which a patient seeks care, the medical diagnosis, is centrally located on the map as shown in Figure 1.4. However, the central figure may not always contain a medical diagnosis. Sometimes the focus of a visit may be on high-level wellness; for example, when a patient will be seen for a screening examination and the aim is to maintain wellness and prevent problems. In a nursing home, the reason for admission to the nursing home is that patients can no longer take care of themselves at home.

The concept care map diagram is primarily composed of nursing diagnoses resulting from the health state, flowing outward from the central figure like spokes on a wheel. The concept care map diagram focuses strictly on real nursing care problems based on collected data. It does not focus on potential problems. At this stage of care planning, it is most important to recognize major problem areas. You do not have to state the nursing diagnosis yet. Write down your general impressions of the patient after your initial review of data.

Labeling the correct diagnosis is difficult for many students. At this point, it is more important to recognize major problem areas than to worry about the correct nursing diagnostic label. If you recognize that the patient has a major problem breathing, write it down. You are first looking for the big picture. Later, you can look up the correct nursing diagnostic label and decide if the diagnosis should be *Impaired Gas Exchange, Ineffective Airway Clearance,* or *Ineffective Breathing Pattern.* Initially, just write, in whatever words come to mind, what you think are the patient's problems. Recognizing that something is wrong with the patient is more important than applying the correct label. Chapter 3 will expand on step 1 on formulating basic diagrams of problems.

Step 2: Analyze and Categorize Data

In this step, you must analyze and categorize data gathered from the patient's medical records

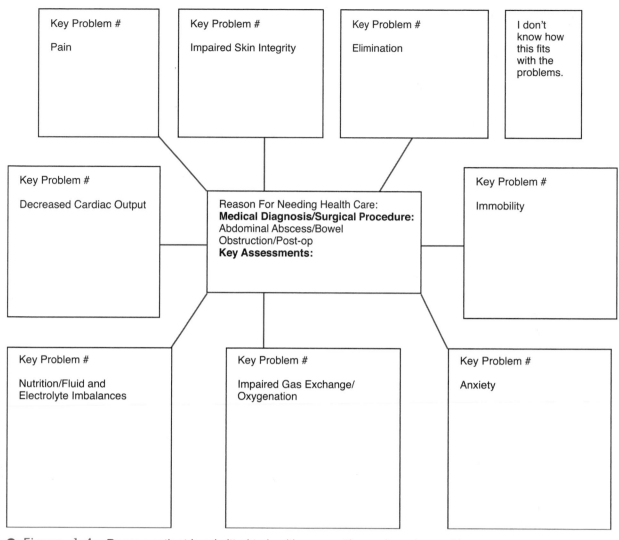

Key Problem #

Pain

Key Problem #

Impaired Skin Integrity

Key Problem #

Elimination

I don't know how this fits with the problems.

Key Problem #

Decreased Cardiac Output

Reason For Needing Health Care:
Medical Diagnosis/Surgical Procedure:
Abdominal Abscess/Bowel Obstruction/Post-op
Key Assessments:

Key Problem #

Immobility

Key Problem #

Nutrition/Fluid and Electrolyte Imbalances

Key Problem #

Impaired Gas Exchange/ Oxygenation

Key Problem #

Anxiety

● Figure 1.4 Reason patient is admitted to health-care setting and nursing problems. Developing the sloppy copy: key ideas based on assessment.

and your brief encounter with the patient. By categorizing the data, you provide evidence to support the medical diagnoses and nursing problems/diagnoses. You must identify and group the most important assessment data related to the patient's reason for seeking health care. You must also identify and group clinical assessment data, pathophysiology, treatments, laboratory data, medications, and medical history data related to the nursing problems/diagnoses, as shown in Figure 1.5.

In this example of a concept care map, you see the nursing problems/diagnoses flowing outward from the patient's reason for seeking health care. Listed under each problem/nursing diagnosis is the clinical evidence that led the creator

of the concept care map to conclude that the problem/diagnosis was appropriate to that patient at that time.

Thus, when making a concept care map, you must write important clinical assessment data, pathophysiology, treatments, laboratory values, medications, and medical history data related to each nursing problem/diagnosis. This involves sifting through and sorting out the often voluminous amount of data that you collected on your patient. The sicker the patient, the more complex the analysis. You need to list assessment data regarding physical and emotional indicators of problems or symptoms of pathology under the appropriate problem/diagnoses. For example, physical indicators include labored respirations

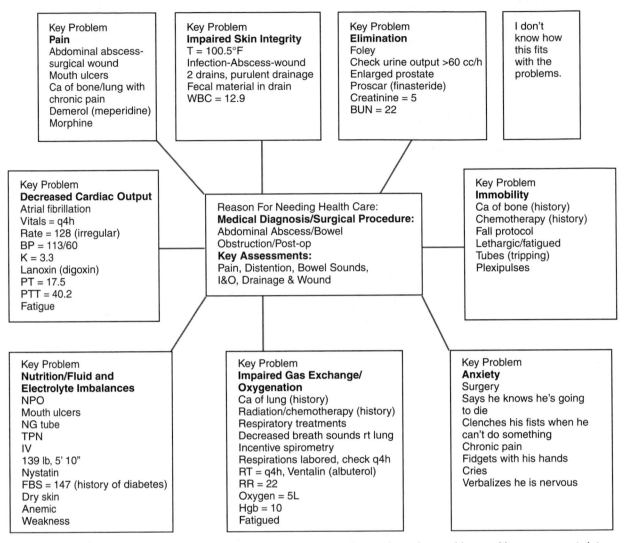

Key Problem
Pain
Abdominal abscess-
surgical wound
Mouth ulcers
Ca of bone/lung with
chronic pain
Demerol (meperidine)
Morphine

Key Problem
Impaired Skin Integrity
T = 100.5°F
Infection-Abscess-wound
2 drains, purulent drainage
Fecal material in drain
WBC = 12.9

Key Problem
Elimination
Foley
Check urine output >60 cc/h
Enlarged prostate
Proscar (finasteride)
Creatinine = 5
BUN = 22

I don't
know how
this fits
with the
problems.

Key Problem
Decreased Cardiac Output
Atrial fibrillation
Vitals = q4h
Rate = 128 (irregular)
BP = 113/60
K = 3.3
Lanoxin (digoxin)
PT = 17.5
PTT = 40.2
Fatigue

Reason For Needing Health Care:
Medical Diagnosis/Surgical Procedure:
Abdominal Abscess/Bowel
Obstruction/Post-op
Key Assessments:
Pain, Distention, Bowel Sounds,
I&O, Drainage & Wound

Key Problem
Immobility
Ca of bone (history)
Chemotherapy (history)
Fall protocol
Lethargic/fatigued
Tubes (tripping)
Plexipulses

Key Problem
**Nutrition/Fluid and
Electrolyte Imbalances**
NPO
Mouth ulcers
NG tube
TPN
IV
139 lb, 5' 10"
Nystatin
FBS = 147 (history of diabetes)
Dry skin
Anemic
Weakness

Key Problem
**Impaired Gas Exchange/
Oxygenation**
Ca of lung (history)
Radiation/chemotherapy (history)
Respiratory treatments
Decreased breath sounds rt lung
Incentive spirometry
Respirations labored, check q4h
RT = q4h, Ventalin (albuterol)
RR = 22
Oxygen = 5L
Hgb = 10
Fatigued

Key Problem
Anxiety
Surgery
Says he knows he's going
to die
Clenches his fists when he
can't do something
Chronic pain
Fidgets with his hands
Cries
Verbalizes he is nervous

● Figure 1.5   Reason patient is admitted to health-care setting and nursing problems with assessment data to support the final edition.

at a rate of 22, fatigue, and decreased breath sounds. These are listed under the nursing diagnosis *Impaired Gas Exchange.* Emotional indicators of problems include the patient crying and verbalizing that he is nervous and saying that he knows he is going to die. These are listed under the nursing diagnosis *Anxiety.* Nursing Diagnoses are italicized and are defined in Appendix C. You must also list current information on diagnostic test data, treatments, and medications under the appropriate nursing diagnoses. You may need to look up the diagnostic tests, treatments, and medications if you are not familiar with them. You must think critically to place diagnostic test

data, treatments, and medications under the appropriate category. For example, diagnostic tests include blood studies of white blood cells, hemoglobin, and potassium. In this case, the white blood cells are listed with *Impaired Skin Integrity* and the abscessed wound; the hemoglobin with *Impaired Gas Exchange,* and the potassium with *Decreased Cardiac Output.* Oxygen and respiratory treatments are categorized with *Impaired Gas Exchange.* The medication morphine is categorized with *Pain;* Ventolin (albuterol) is categorized with *Impaired Gas Exchange;* and Lanoxin (digoxin) is categorized with *Decreased Cardiac Output.*

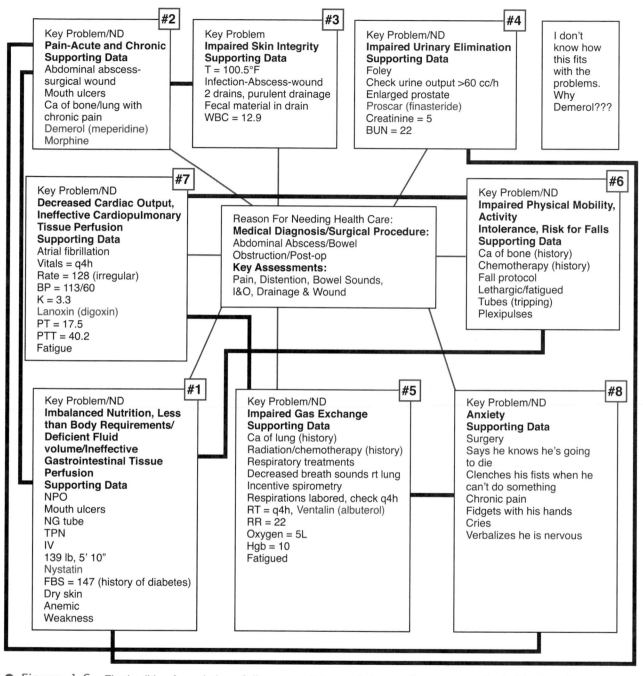

#2
Key Problem/ND
Pain-Acute and Chronic
Supporting Data
Abdominal abscess-
surgical wound
Mouth ulcers
Ca of bone/lung with
chronic pain
Demerol (meperidine)
Morphine

#3
Key Problem
Impaired Skin Integrity
Supporting Data
T = 100.5°F
Infection-Abscess-wound
2 drains, purulent drainage
Fecal material in drain
WBC = 12.9

#4
Key Problem/ND
Impaired Urinary Elimination
Supporting Data
Foley
Check urine output >60 cc/h
Enlarged prostate
Proscar (finasteride)
Creatinine = 5
BUN = 22

I don't
know how
this fits
with the
problems.
Why
Demerol???

#7
Key Problem/ND
Decreased Cardiac Output,
Ineffective Cardiopulmonary
Tissue Perfusion
Supporting Data
Atrial fibrillation
Vitals = q4h
Rate = 128 (irregular)
BP = 113/60
K = 3.3
Lanoxin (digoxin)
PT = 17.5
PTT = 40.2
Fatigue

Reason For Needing Health Care:
Medical Diagnosis/Surgical Procedure:
Abdominal Abscess/Bowel
Obstruction/Post-op
Key Assessments:
Pain, Distention, Bowel Sounds,
I&O, Drainage & Wound

#6
Key Problem/ND
Impaired Physical Mobility,
Activity
Intolerance, Risk for Falls
Supporting Data
Ca of bone (history)
Chemotherapy (history)
Fall protocol
Lethargic/fatigued
Tubes (tripping)
Plexipulses

#1
Key Problem/ND
Imbalanced Nutrition, Less
than Body Requirements/
Deficient Fluid
volume/Ineffective
Gastrointestinal Tissue
Perfusion
Supporting Data
NPO
Mouth ulcers
NG tube
TPN
IV
139 lb, 5' 10"
Nystatin
FBS = 147 (history of diabetes)
Dry skin
Anemic
Weakness

#5
Key Problem/ND
Impaired Gas Exchange
Supporting Data
Ca of lung (history)
Radiation/chemotherapy (history)
Respiratory treatments
Decreased breath sounds rt lung
Incentive spirometry
Respirations labored, check q4h
RT = q4h, Ventalin (albuterol)
RR = 22
Oxygen = 5L
Hgb = 10
Fatigued

#8
Key Problem/ND
Anxiety
Supporting Data
Surgery
Says he knows he's going
to die
Clenches his fists when he
can't do something
Chronic pain
Fidgets with his hands
Cries
Verbalizes he is nervous

● Figure 1.6 Final edition formulation of diagnoses, linkages between diagnoses, and prioritization of problems.

You must also list medical history information under the nursing diagnoses. In this example, the patient has a history of bone and lung cancer, atrial fibrillation, and an enlarged prostate. The bone and lung cancer history is listed under the nursing diagnoses of *Pain,*

Impaired Gas Exchange, and *Impaired Physical Mobility;* atrial fibrillation is under *Decreased Cardiac Output;* and the enlarged prostate is listed under *Impaired Urinary Elimination.*

When beginning to use concept care maps with medical and nursing diagnoses that are new to you, you may not always know where to categorize an abnormal symptom, laboratory value, treatment, drug, or history information. If you do not know where such information should go, list it in the "I don't know how this fits the problem" box of the template, and ask for clarification from your clinical faculty. At least you recognized the information was important; even if you do not yet have the experience to see where the data fit in the overall clinical picture of patient care.

Sometimes you may think that symptoms apply to more than one nursing diagnosis, and they often do. You may recognize that the patient is lethargic and fatigued, but that observation could go under *Decreased Cardiac Output, Impaired Physical Mobility, Imbalanced Nutrition,* or *Impaired Gas Exchange.* It makes sense to place this symptom in more than one area. Therefore, you can repeat a symptom in different categories if it is relevant to more than one category.

Finally, you must determine the priority assessments that still need to be performed regarding the primary reason for seeking care; write them in the box at the center of the map under "Key assessment" in Figure 1.5. In deciding what are the key assessments, consider what would be most the important assessments if you were responsible for assessing a group of six to eight patients, as you will one day as a nurse. These priority assessments must be done on first contact with the patient and carefully monitored throughout the clinical day. Focus on the key areas of physical assessment that must be performed to ensure that the patient's physical problem, which is the reason for admission to the setting, resolves as expected, and intervene immediately with symptoms that indicate complications. This step in the concept care mapping process appears in detail in Chapter 3.

Step 3: Labeling and Analyzing Nursing Diagnoses Relationships

Next, you need to label nursing diagnoses and to analyze relationships among the nursing diagnoses as shown in Figure 1.5. Use Appendixes A to D at the back of the book to find the appropriate label for the diagnosis. Appendixes A, B, and C are classifications of the Nursing Diagnoses according to Maslow (A), Gordon (B), and Doenges (C). Appendix D (NANDA) contains an

alphabetical listing of the nursing diagnoses. Appendix D may help determine the category dealing with respiratory and breathing problems that should be labeled *Impaired Gas Exchange, Ineffective Airway Clearance,* or *Ineffective Cardiopulmonary Tissue Perfusion.*

You will need to prioritize your nursing diagnoses by numbering them. Your priorities are going to be what you think are the most important problems. All the problems you have identified are important, but attempt to number them. Priorities do change throughout the clinical day. You may do the sloppy copy thinking that *Pain* is going to be a top priority, but it turns out that your patient does not have any, and for him *Anxiety* is the major problem of the day. Therefore, use your sloppy copy to guess at the order of priority, but then use your final edition to prioritize accurately what happened during the clinical day.

You will also be drawing lines between nursing diagnoses to indicate relationships as shown in Figure 1.6. In this example, *Pain* is related to *Anxiety, Impaired Physical Mobility, Skin Integrity,* and *Imbalanced Nutrition.* Be prepared to explain to your clinical faculty why you have made these links. You may want to add the words that describe the relationship linkages. For example, why pain and nutrition? In this case, the explanation is that the patient has mouth ulcers and an uncomfortable nasogastric tube, both of which contribute to pain. You will soon recognize that all the problems the patient is having are interrelated. You and your clinical faculty can see the "whole picture" of what is happening with the patient by looking at the map. Thus, concept care maps are a holistic approach to patient care. These issues will be expanded in Chapter 3.

Step 4: Identifying Goals, Outcomes, and Interventions

On the template in Figure 1.7, you will write patient goals and outcomes and then list nursing interventions to attain the outcomes for each of the numbered diagnoses on your concept care map. Outcomes are at the top of the template, with interventions listed in the first column, and goals listed throughout (see Fig. 1.7). You must list the nursing care you intend to provide for the patient during the time that you are scheduled to be interacting with the patient.

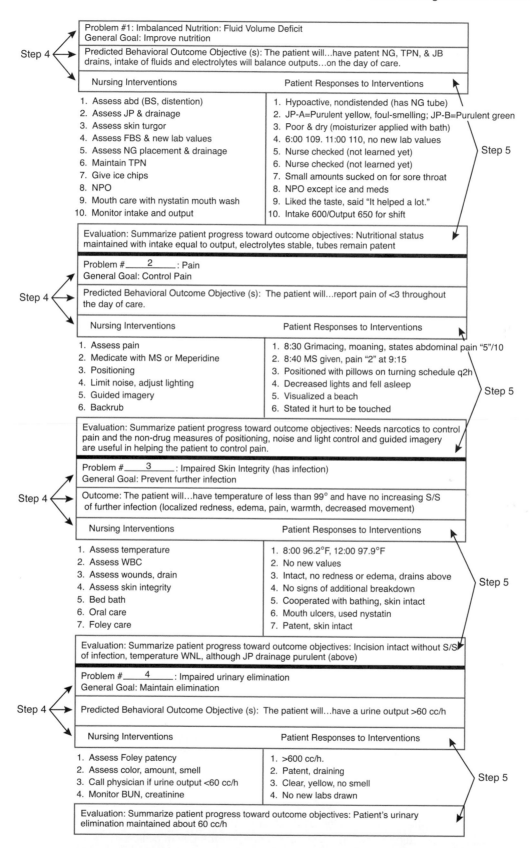

Step 4 →

Problem #1: Imbalanced Nutrition: Fluid Volume Deficit
General Goal: Improve nutrition

Predicted Behavioral Outcome Objective (s): The patient will...have patent NG, TPN, & JB drains, intake of fluids and electrolytes will balance outputs...on the day of care.

Nursing Interventions	Patient Responses to Interventions
1. Assess abd (BS, distention)	1. Hypoactive, nondistended (has NG tube)
2. Assess JP & drainage	2. JP-A=Purulent yellow, foul-smelling; JP-B=Purulent green
3. Assess skin turgor	3. Poor & dry (moisturizer applied with bath)
4. Assess FBS & new lab values	4. 6:00 109. 11:00 110, no new lab values
5. Assess NG placement & drainage	5. Nurse checked (not learned yet)
6. Maintain TPN	6. Nurse checked (not learned yet)
7. Give ice chips	7. Small amounts sucked on for sore throat
8. NPO	8. NPO except ice and meds
9. Mouth care with nystatin mouth wash	9. Liked the taste, said "It helped a lot."
10. Monitor intake and output	10. Intake 600/Output 650 for shift

Step 5

Evaluation: Summarize patient progress toward outcome objectives: Nutritional status maintained with intake equal to output, electrolytes stable, tubes remain patent

Step 4 →

Problem #___2___ : Pain
General Goal: Control Pain

Predicted Behavioral Outcome Objective (s): The patient will...report pain of <3 throughout the day of care.

Nursing Interventions	Patient Responses to Interventions
1. Assess pain	1. 8:30 Grimacing, moaning, states abdominal pain "5"/10
2. Medicate with MS or Meperidine	2. 8:40 MS given, pain "2" at 9:15
3. Positioning	3. Positioned with pillows on turning schedule q2h
4. Limit noise, adjust lighting	4. Decreased lights and fell asleep
5. Guided imagery	5. Visualized a beach
6. Backrub	6. Stated it hurt to be touched

Step 5

Evaluation: Summarize patient progress toward outcome objectives: Needs narcotics to control pain and the non-drug measures of positioning, noise and light control and guided imagery are useful in helping the patient to control pain.

Step 4 →

Problem #___3___ : Impaired Skin Integrity (has infection)
General Goal: Prevent further infection

Outcome: The patient will...have temperature of less than 99° and have no increasing S/S of further infection (localized redness, edema, pain, warmth, decreased movement)

Nursing Interventions	Patient Responses to Interventions
1. Assess temperature	1. 8:00 96.2°F, 12:00 97.9°F
2. Assess WBC	2. No new values
3. Assess wounds, drain	3. Intact, no redness or edema, drains above
4. Assess skin integrity	4. No signs of additional breakdown
5. Bed bath	5. Cooperated with bathing, skin intact
6. Oral care	6. Mouth ulcers, used nystatin
7. Foley care	7. Patent, skin intact

Step 5

Evaluation: Summarize patient progress toward outcome objectives: Incision intact without S/S of infection, temperature WNL, although JP drainage purulent (above)

Step 4 →

Problem #___4___ : Impaired urinary elimination
General Goal: Maintain elimination

Predicted Behavioral Outcome Objective (s): The patient will...have a urine output >60 cc/h

Nursing Interventions	Patient Responses to Interventions
1. Assess Foley patency	1. >600 cc/h.
2. Assess color, amount, smell	2. Patent, draining
3. Call physician if urine output <60 cc/h	3. Clear, yellow, no smell
4. Monitor BUN, creatinine	4. No new labs drawn

Step 5

Evaluation: Summarize patient progress toward outcome objectives: Patient's urinary elimination maintained about 60 cc/h

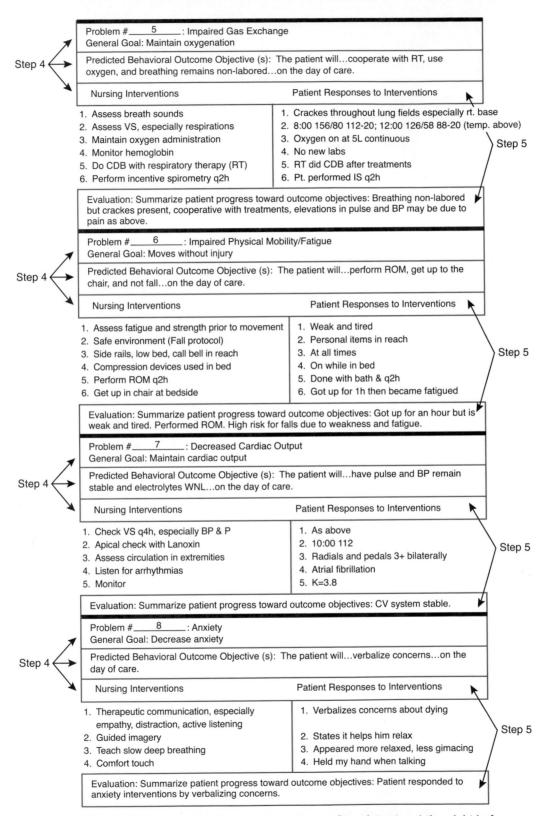

Problem #_____5_____: Impaired Gas Exchange
General Goal: Maintain oxygenation

Step 4

Predicted Behavioral Outcome Objective (s): The patient will...cooperate with RT, use oxygen, and breathing remains non-labored...on the day of care.

Nursing Interventions	Patient Responses to Interventions
1. Assess breath sounds	1. Crackes throughout lung fields especially rt. base
2. Assess VS, especially respirations	2. 8:00 156/80 112-20; 12:00 126/58 88-20 (temp. above)
3. Maintain oxygen administration	3. Oxygen on at 5L continuous
4. Monitor hemoglobin	4. No new labs
5. Do CDB with respiratory therapy (RT)	5. RT did CDB after treatments
6. Perform incentive spirometry q2h	6. Pt. performed IS q2h

Step 5

Evaluation: Summarize patient progress toward outcome objectives: Breathing non-labored but crackes present, cooperative with treatments, elevations in pulse and BP may be due to pain as above.

Problem #_____6_____: Impaired Physical Mobility/Fatigue
General Goal: Moves without injury

Step 4

Predicted Behavioral Outcome Objective (s): The patient will...perform ROM, get up to the chair, and not fall...on the day of care.

Nursing Interventions	Patient Responses to Interventions
1. Assess fatigue and strength prior to movement	1. Weak and tired
2. Safe environment (Fall protocol)	2. Personal items in reach
3. Side rails, low bed, call bell in reach	3. At all times
4. Compression devices used in bed	4. On while in bed
5. Perform ROM q2h	5. Done with bath & q2h
6. Get up in chair at bedside	6. Got up for 1h then became fatigued

Step 5

Evaluation: Summarize patient progress toward outcome objectives: Got up for an hour but is weak and tired. Performed ROM. High risk for falls due to weakness and fatigue.

Problem #_____7_____: Decreased Cardiac Output
General Goal: Maintain cardiac output

Step 4

Predicted Behavioral Outcome Objective (s): The patient will...have pulse and BP remain stable and electrolytes WNL...on the day of care.

Nursing Interventions	Patient Responses to Interventions
1. Check VS q4h, especially BP & P	1. As above
2. Apical check with Lanoxin	2. 10:00 112
3. Assess circulation in extremities	3. Radials and pedals 3+ bilaterally
4. Listen for arrhythmias	4. Atrial fibrillation
5. Monitor	5. K=3.8

Step 5

Evaluation: Summarize patient progress toward outcome objectives: CV system stable.

Problem #_____8_____: Anxiety
General Goal: Decrease anxiety

Step 4

Predicted Behavioral Outcome Objective (s): The patient will...verbalize concerns...on the day of care.

Nursing Interventions	Patient Responses to Interventions
1. Therapeutic communication, especially empathy, distraction, active listening	1. Verbalizes concerns about dying
2. Guided imagery	2. States it helps him relax
3. Teach slow deep breathing	3. Appeared more relaxed, less gimacing
4. Comfort touch	4. Held my hand when talking

Step 5

Evaluation: Summarize patient progress toward outcome objectives: Patient responded to anxiety interventions by verbalizing concerns.

● Figure 1.7   Steps 4 and 5 of the concept care map. Complete step 4 the night before clinical. Step 5: Evaluation of patient responses. Complete the day of clinical.

You will carry the sloppy copy care map, goals, outcomes, and intervention lists in your pocket as you work with the patient, and you will either check off interventions as you complete them or make revisions in the diagram and interventions as you interact with the patient. The concept care maps with interventions are used during the intervention phase of the nursing process.

The nursing interventions include key areas of assessment and monitoring as well as procedures or other therapeutic interventions such as patient teaching or therapeutic communication. To decrease paperwork, rationales for interventions are not written down. Come prepared to explain verbally the rationales for your identified nursing interventions if asked by your clinical faculty. It is of course a professional responsibility to know why you are doing each action, even though you are not writing it down.

Be prepared to review nursing interventions during clinical preconferencing. Nursing interventions include what you are supposed to be monitoring carefully. In addition, nursing interventions should include a list of all appropriate treatments and medications. Patient teaching should be listed under nursing interventions as appropriate for each problem. For example, patient teaching may involve slow, deep breathing and guided imagery under the nursing diagnosis *Anxiety*.

If you have not yet learned how to perform a treatment but you know the treatment needs to be done to address a problem, list it in the nursing intervention column, and also note that the nurse assigned to oversee the patient's care will be doing the treatment. For example, under *Imbalanced Nutrition*, you may write that the patient needs total parenteral nutrition and care of the nasogastric tube but that these services will be done by the staff nurse because you have not yet learned how to provide them. By recording the treatments in the appropriate column, you demonstrate that you have recognized these nutrition-related treatments and that they are important aspects of the total care needed by the patient. Be prepared to discuss the basic purpose of the interventions, even those you do not perform yourself. Chapter 4 will expand on step 4 outcomes and nursing interventions.

Step 5: **Evaluate Patient's Responses**

This step is the written evaluation of the patient's physical and psychosocial responses. It is shown in the second column of Figure 1.7. As you perform a nursing activity, record the patient's responses. For example, you said that you would monitor the patient's temperature in step 4 under the nursing diagnosis *Impaired Skin Integrity*. In step 5, you record those temperatures across from the intervention. Step 5 also involves writing your clinical impressions and inferences regarding the patient's progress toward expected outcomes and the effectiveness of your interventions to bring these outcomes about. This is an evaluation statement written to summarize progress toward the outcome objectives for each nursing diagnosis, found at the beginning of each intervention and response list. Step 5 on evaluation of outcomes will be expanded in Chapters 5 and 6.

During Clinical Care: Keep It in Your Pocket

Throughout the clinical day, you and your clinical faculty will have an ongoing discussion regarding changes in patient assessment data, effectiveness of interventions, and patient responses to those interventions. Keep the concept care map in your pocket; this way, everything that must be done and evaluated is listed succinctly and kept within easy reach. As the plan is revised throughout the day, take notes on the concept care map diagram, add or delete nursing interventions, and write patient responses as you go along. As your clinical faculty makes rounds and checks in on you and your patients, the faculty can also refer to the concept care maps with goals, outcomes, and interventions you have developed as the basis for guiding your patient care.

Documentation

The concept care maps with interventions and patient responses will become the basis of your documentation. You will be using the revised plans and outcome evaluations as guides to make sure you have documented patient problems, interventions, and the evaluation of patient responses adequately. Documentation involves correctly identifying patient assessment data to record a problem, determining what to record about the interventions to correct the problem, and describing the patient's responses to the interventions. Assessment, interventions, and responses are all present in the concept care map. Concept care maps as the basis of documentation will be described in more detail in Chapter 7.

Medication Administration

Your concept care map will also be useful as you prepare to administer medications. By organizing the drugs to be administered under the correct problem, you demonstrate your knowledge of the relationship of the drug to the problem. You can also see the interactive effects of the drug related to the total clinical picture. For example, as you discuss Lanoxin (digitalis) administration under *Decreased Cardiac Output,* you and your clinical faculty can also see that the patient's potassium level was low. What is the relationship between low levels of potassium and Lanoxin administration? The answer is an increased risk of a toxic reaction by the patient to digitalis. Be prepared for your clinical faculty to ask you for the current value of potassium from the morning blood draw. Low potassium levels have to be corrected; in the meantime, you can be assessing the patient carefully for adverse reactions to the drug. You can more easily integrate medications with laboratory values and pathology if the information is all neatly categorized under *Decreased Cardiac Output.*

In addition, you should also record scheduled times of medication administration next to the drugs. You may also highlight drugs on the map. Writing down administration times and highlighting drugs help to organize and remind you of the importance of the medication administration times. It also decreases the chance of medication errors.

Nursing Standards of Care

Concept care maps are individualized plans of care built on critical analysis of patient assessment data, identification of medical and nursing diagnoses, determination of nursing actions to be implemented, and evaluation of patient responses. Development, implementation, and evaluation of safe and effective nursing care are contingent upon nurses knowing and following accepted standards of care. As you plan care for a patient, a primary question you must address is: What are the standards of care pertinent to my patient and specific to the applicable medical and nursing diagnoses? Nursing students often wonder: "Have I included everything necessary in this care plan?," "Am I doing everything I should be doing?," "Am I missing something?" Following standards of care ensures that you are doing everything possible to provide appropriate care to the patient. These standards may stem from several organizing agencies or principles.

Standards of the ANA

By law, nurses must follow guidelines for the safe and effective practice of nursing. These legal guidelines are called *standards of care.* The ANA has developed general standards of nursing practice, shown in Box 1.1.[17] Concept care maps are in compliance with these general standards of care.

Standards of the Joint Commission on Accreditation of Health Care Organizations

The Joint Commission on Accreditation of Health Care Organizations (JCAHO) provides very specific standards to be followed for nursing care for patients. JCAHO requires that all accredited agencies have written policies and procedures for nursing care. You must follow these specific policies and procedures for any nursing care you administer. Representatives of JCAHO travel the country and review these policies and procedures. If they are not current, JCAHO requires that they be updated if the agency desires to maintain its certification.

Fortunately for you as a student, fundamentals and medical-surgical textbooks provide general descriptions of procedures similar to what is required by your clinical agency. Your clinical faculty will inform you of any specific require-

Box 1.1	ANA STANDARDS OF NURSING PRACTICE

1. The collection of data about the health status of the client/patient is systematic and continuous. The data are accessible, communicated, and recorded.
2. Nursing diagnoses are derived from health status data.
3. The plan of care includes goals derived from the nursing diagnoses.
4. The plan of nursing care includes the priorities and the prescribed nursing approaches or measures to achieve the goals derived from the diagnoses.
5. Nursing actions provide for client/patient participation and health promotions, maintenance, and restoration.
6. Nursing actions assist the client/patient to maximize his health capabilities.
7. The client's/patient's progress or lack of progress toward goal achievement is determined by the client/patient and the nurse.
8. The client's/patient's progress or lack of progress toward goal achievement directs reassessment, reordering of priorities, new goal setting, and revision of the plan of nursing care.

Nursing's Social Policy Statement, ed 2. American Nurses Association, Washington, D.C., 2003.

ments of the clinical agency in which you are placed, either by explaining those requirements verbally or referring you to the agency's procedure manual.

Standardized Nursing Care Plans

Many organizations have developed standardized nursing care plans for specific medical diagnoses. These standardized nursing care plans are based on typical nursing diagnoses of patients with particular medical problems. Many facilities have general nursing care plans for nursing care of patients who are commonly seen. For example, an orthopedic unit probably has a standardized care plan for the patient with a fractured hip, and the urology unit probably has a standardized care plan for the patient undergoing a transurethral resection of the prostate gland. In addition, hundreds of standardized care plans have been written and published, and many have been computerized for easy accessibility.

Therefore, while you are gathering data from a patient's records to prepare your care map, you also need to find out whether the agency has any standardized care plans available for you to use. If these plans are not available on the unit to which you are assigned, you can use published standardized care plan books to make sure you have not missed any important aspects of care.

Patient Education Standards

All patients have the right to know what is wrong with them and how to manage their own care. That makes patient education a key role for nurses. Most agencies have patient education materials available that are specific to various types of problems. You also need to collect these materials when you collect information from patient records. As with standardized care plans, standardized teaching materials, such as booklets and movies, have been published that may be available for you and the patient as references. Teaching materials are usually geared toward a fifth-grade reading level. Materials given to patients must be carefully screened for content that is appropriate for the patient's individual needs and ability to comprehend the materials. Detailed information about integrating teaching materials with care maps appears in later chapters.

Insurance Agency and Government Care Standards

The high cost of health care has led to a concerted effort by the government (which pays for Medicare and Medicaid) and health-care insurance companies to control costs. At the same time that costs are being controlled, the quality of health care is supposed to be ensured through careful management by health-care providers. The government and insurance companies have developed specific criteria for which services will and will not be reimbursed, depending on diagnoses. All medications, treatments, surgeries, and rehabilitation programs (literally everything done by health-care providers) have to be provided and documented according to government and insurance company criteria for care, or the bills will not be paid. When bills are not paid by the government or insurance companies, health-care providers may never receive payment for services provided. In some cases, patients may be left with the bill. In that case, patients may decide to go without needed health-care services because they cannot afford them.

Insurance companies and the government pay predetermined amounts of money to agencies or physicians providing care to patients. For example, if a patient has knee replacement surgery, the providers will receive a fixed amount of money for that service. Case managers, typically advanced practice nurses, are hired by insurance companies and health-care agencies to evaluate the types of care given to inpatients and outpatients, to monitor patient progress, and to coordinate the care of patients to guide their recovery while minimizing costs. These case managers are also known as resource managers because they coordinate all services available to the patient. They must be aware of all resources available so they can make the appropriate linkages between patients and the appropriate services.

Teams of health-care providers, including physicians, nurses, pharmacists, dietitians, physical therapists, and social workers, have developed standards that guide the treatment of patients. Instead of separate plans of care from the physician, dietitian, and others, the trend is for health-care providers to collaborate and develop one unified plan of care. This multidisciplinary plan is commonly called a *clinical pathway* or a *critical pathway*. There is careful sequencing of clinical interventions over a specific period that all involved in the care of the patient agree to follow. Clinical pathways outline assessments, treatments, procedures, diet, activities, patient education, and discharge planning activities. Although clinical pathways are becoming a popular method of collaborative care planning, they are not available for every diagnosis. Clinical pathways also vary slightly among clinical agencies.

As you prepare for a clinical care assignment, it is important that you know about the clinical pathway your patient is supposed to be following based on the patient's health condition. Because nurses often spend more time with patients than other health-care providers, nurses' clinical roles include communicating between caregivers to make sure that the patient is making steady progress in the expected direction toward health goals enumerated on the clinical pathway. The nursing care plan and assessment are focused on identifying complications and intervening quickly to get the patient back on the clinical pathway to resume rapid progress toward health goals.

Currently, a battle is raging between health-care providers and those who pay the bills for services, namely the government (for Medicare and Medicaid) and the insurance companies. At one time, physicians ordered whichever tests they believed necessary to diagnose problems and whichever treatments they deemed necessary to fix those problems. If a physician thought that a patient would benefit from an extra day in the hospital, the patient stayed in the hospital. If the physician ordered certain medications to treat the patient's problem, the patient received them. Now, physicians have been forced to use criteria established by insurance companies and the government for diagnosing, treating, admitting, and discharging patients—or the bill is not paid. In essence, the view of the insurance company and government is that physicians are free to treat patients as they deem necessary. But if physicians deviate from the established standards and criteria for treatment, they are not paid. A few years ago, the standard used by those paying the bills was that patients were required to leave the hospital 24 hours after vaginal childbirth. The outcry from the public and from health-care providers grew so loud that the length of stay for vaginal delivery has now increased to 48 hours. But 20 years ago, a woman stayed in the hospital for 4 or 5 days after such a delivery.

Although this is a simple explanation of the current state of affairs regarding payment for services and maintaining quality of care, it is a very complex problem. The complexity exists because the government and insurance agencies differ in types of payment plans and criteria that form the standards of care. In addition, the criteria are under constant revision.

Utilization Review Standards

Documentation of detailed assessments, accuracy of diagnoses, and appropriateness of treatments and follow-up are constantly being reviewed in all health-care settings (such as private physicians' offices, outpatient facilities, and hospitals). Everything and everyone is under *utilization review*—the process of evaluating care given by nurses and physicians and all other health-care providers and agencies. Nurses, primarily, manage utilization reviews, armed with specific criteria for auditing individual health-care providers and the delivery of services in each health-care setting. These nurses are hired by health-care agencies and by insurance companies. Utilization reviewers do not usually have direct contact with patients; they review charts only. They judge the necessity and appropriateness of care and the efficiency with which care is delivered.

Managed Care in Hospital Settings

There is a direct relationship between the care standards described above and the management of care. Currently, nearly all patients who enter hospitals find themselves in managed-care delivery systems. Typically, patients entering health-care facilities have nurse case managers assigned to monitor and coordinate their progress through the system. These case managers are experienced nurses, most of them holding advanced degrees or specialty certifications. These nurses manage hospital resources carefully and coordinate discharge planning. With strict criteria imposed by government and insurance agencies to ensure rapid discharge from acute care facilities, all nurses must carefully document and justify complications and additional problems with patients to ensure that quality care is rendered and financial obligations are met (that is, the bills are paid by government and insurance agencies). These nurses monitor patient progress, and especially track high-risk patients, as well as all patients with complications. These hospital-based nurse case managers interact with service providers and with insurance providers; thus, they are considered resource managers. It is essential to make links for patients to home health services, transitional care units, long-term care facilities, and other agencies to provide quality care.

CHAPTER 1 SUMMARY

The purposes of concept care maps include assisting you with critical thinking, analyzing clinical data, and planning comprehensive nursing care for your patients. A concept care map is based on theories of learning and educational psychology and is a diagrammatic teaching/learning strategy that provides the opportunity to visualize interrelationships between medical and nursing diagnoses, assessment data, and treatments. The visual diagram and interventions are personal pocket guides to patient care, and they form the basis for discussion of nursing care between you and your clinical faculty.

Before developing a concept care map, you must perform a comprehensive patient assessment. Then, in step 1 of concept care mapping, you develop a skeleton diagram of health problems. In step 2, you analyze and categorize specific patient assessment data. In step 3, you label diagnoses, prioritize, and indicate relationships between nursing and medical diagnoses. In step 4, you develop patient goals, outcomes, and nursing interventions for each nursing diagnosis. In step 5, you evaluate the patient's response to each specific nursing intervention and summarize your clinical impressions.

The development of concept care maps is based on understanding and integrating accepted standards of patient care. Standards of care are derived from the standards of the ANA, JCAHO, standard nursing care plans, standards of patient teaching, clinical pathways, insurance agency and government payment standards, and utilization review standards. As a result of these standards, hospitals have become centers for managed care and are employing nursing case managers as patient care resource coordinators. All parties involved with health-care delivery, including health-care agencies and providers, insurance companies, and the government, are finding ways to decrease costs while attempting to maintain quality services through managed care.

LEARNING ACTIVITIES

1. Identify the names and locations of books and computer software that contain standardized nursing care plans that you can use as resources for patient care.

2. Locate samples of standards of care at your assigned clinical agency. Bring to class for discussion a standard nursing care plan from a local agency, a clinical pathway, a standardized specific procedure, and patient education materials.

3. Locate the procedure manual from a local health-care agency, and compare a procedure you are currently learning from your procedures text with the same procedure in the agency's manual.

4. Identify the person or people at your agency who perform case management, discharge planning, and utilization review. Invite one of them to a clinical post-conference to describe his or her role in decreasing costs while maintaining quality of care in the managed care environment.

REFERENCES

1. Schuster, PM: Concept maps: Reducing clinical care plan paperwork and increasing learning. Nurse Educator 25(2):76, 2000.
2. Novak, J, and Gowin, DB: Learning How to Learn. Cambridge University Press, New York, 1984.
3. Ausubel, DP, Novak, JD, and Hanesian, H: Educational Psychology: A Cognitive View, ed 2. Werbel and Peck, New York, 1986.
4. Worrell, P: Metacognition: Implications for instruction in nursing education. J Nurs Educ 29(4):170, 1990.
5. All, AC, and Havens, RL: Cognitive/ concept map: A teaching strategy for nursing. J Adv Nurs 25:1210, 1997.
6. Baugh, NG, and Mellott, KG: Clinical concept maps as preparation for student nurses' clinical experiences. J Nurs Educ 37(6):253, 1998.
7. Daley, BJ, et al: Concept maps: A strategy to teach and evaluate critical thinking. J Nurs Educ 38(1):42, 1999.
8. Daley, B: Concept maps: Linking nursing theory to clinical nursing practice. Journal of Continuing Education in Nursing 27(1):17, 1996.
9. Irvine, L: Can concept maps be used to promote meaningful learning in nurse education? J Adv Nurs 21:1175, 1995.
10. Kathol, DD, et al: Clinical correlation map: A tool for linking theory and practice. Nurse Educator 23(4):31, 1998.
11. Novak, J, and Gowin, DB: op cit.
12. Ausubel, DP, et al: op cit.
13. American Philosophical Association. Critical thinking: A statement of expert consensus for purposes of educational assessment and instruction. Center on

Education and Training for Employ-
ment, College of Education, The Ohio
State University. (ERIC Document
Reproduction No. ED 315-423) Colum-
bus, OH, 1990.

14. McDonald, M: Critical thinking.
National League for Nursing Assessment and Evaluation Quarterly 1(3),
2000.

15. Schuster, P: Concept maps in clinical
settings: Improved clinical performance
and effective patient care. Dean's Notes
25(2), 2003.

16. Nursing's social policy statement, ed 2.
American Nurses Association, Washington, D.C., 2003.

17. Nursing's social policy statement, ed 2.
op cit.

GATHERING CLINICAL DATA:
The Foundation for the Concept Care Maps

OBJECTIVES

1. Identify nursing standards of care for systematically gathering clinical data to construct a basic patient profile database.

2. Describe essential components of a basic patient profile database that are needed to develop a concept care map.

3. Explain the purpose of each component of the basic patient profile database.

4. Identify where to search for clinical data in health-care agencies to develop basic patient profile databases.

5. Identify standardized forms to obtain from the agency relevant to a concept care map.

6. Describe how to communicate with staff in the agency when you cannot find clinical data.

Gathering assessment data is the most important thing that student nurses do. This is because each decision regarding patient care is based on clinical data. Sound clinical judgments are based on accurate and complete data collection. The best nurses are excellent at assessment and know why each piece of assessment data is important to the clinical picture.

Many nursing students feel overwhelmed trying to collect relevant clinical data for their first patient assignments when they arrive at a new clinical unit or agency. These same feelings occur each time the student moves to a new agency. As a matter of fact, even experienced nurses feel intimidated by moving from a familiar agency or unit to a new clinical setting, because they fear they may miss important symptoms that will hinder their ability to make sound clinical judgments.

The purpose of this chapter is to give you guidelines for collecting relevant clinical data based on standards of nursing care. Nursing students are sometimes confused about what is and what is not important clinical data. Therefore, the chapter will describe the reasons why each piece of data is needed, along with where to look for the information in order to develop a plan of care that is a concept care map. In addition, the chapter outlines the important skill of communicating effectively with staff when you cannot find the information you need to develop a plan of care.

Standards of Care: Accountability and Responsibility

Nursing students learn early in their nursing programs that they must be accountable and responsible. That is, student nurses are responsible for the nursing care they administer to their assigned patients. Student nurses must account for their clinical performance to clinical faculty, who are responsible and accountable for each student. In a clinical agency, the faculty accounts primarily to the nursing manager regarding student activities related to caring for patients. The nurse manager oversees the provision of nursing care.

In addition to being accountable to faculty, students work directly with and are accountable to agency staff nurses. Agency nurses are responsible for overseeing the care of your patients, and they report directly to the nursing manager. You must know who the staff nurse is for your patient at all times and keep this nurse and your clinical faculty informed of current assessment information. You must tell this nurse the interventions you will and will not be able to provide to the patient. You must never leave patients for a break or for any other reason without giving the staff nurses and your clinical faculty the most recent assessment data for your assigned patients. Communication between you, your faculty, and the staff nurse who is responsible for your assigned patient is critical for safe nursing care of patients.

Student nurses, clinical faculty, and the nursing staff at each agency are legally responsi-

ble and accountable. Professional nurses and student nurses may be taken to court and prosecuted for acting in an irresponsible manner. This may sound threatening, but professional nurses and student nurses are responsible and accountable for the care of human beings. Nursing care of patients involves awesome responsibility with possible legal consequences for negligence or recklessness when performing outside the standards of care.

Standards of care are inextricably linked to professional accountability and responsibility. You, your faculty, and staff nurses must follow standards of care to act accountably and responsibly. The complete listing of the standards of care are listed in Chapter 1 in Box 1.1. For purposes of this chapter, we will focus on the American Nurses Association (ANA) first standard of practice. This standard involves the collection of data. Specifically, the ANA states that collection of data about a patient's health status is to be systematic and continuous and that data must be accessible, recorded, and communicated.[1] The Joint Commission on Accreditation of Healthcare Organizations (JCAHO) also upholds this same standard.

Data collection occurs *before* development of a plan of care, *before* implementation of nursing care, *during* implementation of nursing care, and *during* evaluation of the patient; therefore, it is continuous. All data must be entered on patient records and be accessible to all healthcare providers. The frustrating problem for many students is that they do not know where to look for data in a clinical area. Furthermore, especially early in nursing education, students typically do not know the most important data to collect. Sometimes students cannot read the writing or understand the abbreviations. Keep in mind that the information exists; you just have to find it. According to ANA Standard 1, data must be accessible and recorded. Once you have found the information, of course, you have to know what it means and why it is important.

Finding Important Data

Students are usually given course assessment guidelines to follow when collecting data on patients. A typical example of a database patient profile is in Figure 2.1. This basic patient profile database has been used to collect data for patients admitted to inpatient or outpatient agencies such as hospitals or outpatient same-day surgical centers. This assessment tool will serve as the basis of the concept map to be discussed in Chapter 3.

You must know the essential components of a basic patient profile database, the purpose of each component of the profile, and where to search for the information in health-care agencies. This database has physical, psychological, social, and cultural components. Most of the information is collected from patient notes and records, and the remainder may be collected from a brief encounter with your patient and a conversation with the patient's assigned agency nurse. It is best if you can obtain your assignment the evening before clinical, because you have more time to think critically and analyze the data you obtained and put together a care plan. In outpatient settings, this may not be possible. Students who are unable to obtain an assignment the day before clinical may have to collect data and develop a care plan on the day of care. Each component of the database will be described carefully in the following sections. Refer to Figure 2.1 as you read the remainder of the chapter. Each component of the patient database in Figure 2.1 has been numbered to correspond with the explanations for each component written in the following sections.

1) Student Name and Date of Care

Your name and date of care are needed to help your clinical faculty keep your database separate from those of the other nursing students at your clinical agency.

2) Patient Initials

Never write a patient's full name on anything that will be taken out of the hospital. All information recorded on the patient profile is confidential. Confidentiality involves ethical and legal standards of care. It is your ethical and legal responsibility to reveal confidential information only to health-care professionals directly involved in the patient's care. Be very careful what you do with confidential information. Never leave forms lying

around in patient rooms where the patient, family, and friends may read what you have written, even if you include only initials on the data. Never discuss data with anyone outside the health-care agency. If a patient's family or friends ask a general question about how the patient is doing, give a general answer, such as "Fine. He's coming along nicely. He ate well, and he's up and moving around" or "Not so good today. He's hurting and tired." Do not reveal the specifics of the diagnosis and prognosis. You should tell the inquiring person that the information is confidential and that he should discuss the specifics directly with the patient or with the physician.

3) Age, Growth, and Development

The patient's age can be obtained from the face sheet of the chart. It is one of the first few sheets that you will find as you open the chart. The face sheet is the page that is typed by the hospital registration department. On entry to the health-care agency, the first stop the patient makes is the registration desk, where the patient (or a family member) registers for admission.

Age is a very important factor to consider. You must be aware of the human growth and developmental tasks across the life span, and then consider how the current health problem has affected the patient's ability to accomplish the developmental tasks at hand. Eric H. Erickson[2] has a widely known theory of eight stages of human growth and development with which you should be familiar.

Stage 1: *Trust Versus Mistrust*

During the first year of life, an infant must learn to trust the people in his environment. When caretakers meet the infant's needs for food, warmth, security, and love, the infant will learn to expect what will happen and can trust those around him to provide what he needs. He feels secure. When an infant's needs are not met, he becomes fearful and mistrusting. Some of these infants fail to thrive. Failure to thrive is a medical diagnosis according to which an infant may fail to gain weight or may even lose it. This problem may stem from such environmental causes as physical starvation or emotional deprivation of love and security.

Student Name:

1) Date of Care:	2) Patient Initials:	3) Age: (face sheet)	3) Growth and Development	4) Gender: (face sheet)	5) Admission Date: (face sheet)

6) Reason for hospitalization (face sheet): Describe reason for hospitalization: (expand on back of page) *Medical Dx:* *Pathophysiology:* *All signs and symptoms: Highlight those your patient exhibits*	7) Chronic illnesses (physician's history and physical notes in chart; nursing intake assessment and Kardex)
8) Surgical procedures (consent forms and Kardex): Describe surgical procedure (expand on back of page) Name of surgical procedure: *Describe surgery:*	

9) ADVANCE DIRECTIVES (NURSE'S ADMISSION ASSESSMENTS):

Living will: ☐ Yes ☐ No	Power of attorney: ☐ Yes ☐ No	Do not resuscitate (DNR) order (Kardex): ☐ Yes ☐ No

10) LABORATORY DATA:

Test	Normal Values	Admission	Date/Time	Date/Time	Reason for Abnormal Values
White blood cells (WBCs)					
Red blood cells (RBCs)					
Hemoglobin (Hgb)					
Hematocrit (Hct)					
Platelets					
Prothrombin time (PT)					
International normalized ratio (INR)					
Activated partial thromboplastin time (Aptt)					
Sodium Na					
Potassium K					
Chloride Cl					
Glucose (FBS/BS)					
Hemoglobin A1C					
Cholesterol					
Blood Urea Nitrogen (BUN)					
Creatinine					
Urine analysis (UA)					
Pre-albumin					
Albumin					
Calcium Ca					
Phosphate					
Bilirubin					
Alkaline phosphatase					
SGOT-Serum glutamic-oxyloacetic transaminase					
AST-Serum glutamic pyruvic transaminase					
CK					
CK MB					
Troponin					
B-natriuretic peptide BNP					
pH					
pCO_2					
pO_2					
HCO_3					

11) DIAGNOSTIC TESTS

Chest x-ray:	EKG:	Other abnormal reports:
Sputum or Blood Culture:	Other:	Other:

12) MEDICATIONS   List medications and times of administration (medication administration record and check the drawer in the carts for spelling). Include over-the-counter (OTC) products/herbal medicines.

Times Due				
Brand Name				
Generic Name				
Dose				
Administration Route				
Classification				
Action				
Reason This Patient is Receiving				
Pharmacokinetics	O P D 1/2 M E	O P D 1/2 M E	O P D 1/2 M E	O P D 1/2 M E
Contraindications				
Major Adverse Side Effects				
Nursing Implications				
Pt/Family Teaching				

Developed by P. Testa, YSU

ALLERGIES/PAINS

13) Allergies: Type of Reaction: (medication administration record):	14) When was the last time pain medication given? (medication administration record)
14) Where is the pain? (nurse's notes)	14) How much pain is the patient in on a scale 0-10? (nurse's notes, flow sheet):

TREATMENTS

15) List treatments (Kardex): Rationale for treatments:
Dressing changes Ice Foley NG Position changes q2h Ted Hose SCDs IS q1h while awake C&DB q1h while awake etc.
16) Support services (Kardex) What do support services provide for the patient?
17) What does the consultant do for the patient?:

18) DIET/FLUIDS

Type of Diet (Kardex):	Restrictions (Kardex):	Gag reflex intact: ☐Yes ☐No	Appetite: ☐Good ☐Fair ☐Poor	Breakfast ____ %	Lunch ____ %	Dinner ____ %

What type of diet is this?:
What types of foods are included in this diet and what foods should be avoided?:

Circle Those Problems That Apply:	
Prior 8 hours Fluid intake: (Oral & IV) Fluid output (flow sheet)	• Problems: swallowing, chewing, dentures (nurse's notes) • Needs assistance with feeding (nurse's notes) • Nausea or vomiting (nurse's notes) • Overhydrated or dehydrated (evaluate total intake and output on flow sheet)
Tube feedings: Type and rate (Kardex)	• Belching: • Other: _____

19) INTRAVENOUS FLUIDS (IV therapy record)

Type and Rate:	IV dressing dry, no edema, redness of site: ☐Yes ☐No	Other:

20) ELIMINATION (flow sheet)

Last bowel movement:	Foley/condom catheter: ☐ Yes ☐ No
Circle Those Problems That Apply:	

• Bowel: constipation diarrhea flatus incontinence belching
• Urinary: hesitancy frequency burning incontinence odor
• Other: _____
• What is causing the problem in elimination? _____

21) ACTIVITY (Kardex, flow sheet)

Ability to walk (gait):	Type of activity orders:	Use of assistance devices: cane, walker, crutches, prosthesis:	Falls-risk assessment rating:
No. of side rails required (flow sheet)	Restraints (flow sheet): ☐ Yes ☐ No	Weakness ☐ Yes ☐ No	Trouble sleeping (nurse's notes): ☐ Yes ☐ No

What does activity order mean?: _____
Why isn't the patient up ad lib?: _____
Would the problem cause weakness?: _____

PHYSICAL ASSESSMENT DATA

22) BP (flow sheet):	2) TPR (flow sheet):	23) Height: _____ Weight: _____ (nursing intake assessments)

24) NEUROLOGICAL/MENTAL STATUS:

LOC: alert and oriented to person, place, time (A&O x 3), confused, etc.	Speech: clear, appropriate/inappropriate
Pupils: PERRLA	Sensory deficits for vision/hearing/taste/ smell

25) MUSCULOSKELETAL STATUS:

Bones, joints, muscles (fractures, contractures, arthritis, spinal curvatures, etc):	Extremity (temperature, edema (pitting vs. nonpitting) & sensation)
Motor: ROM x 4 extremities	
Ted hose/plexi pulses/compression devices: type:	Casts, splint, collar, brace:

26) CARDIOVASCULAR SYSTEM:

Pulses (radial, pedal) (to touch or with Doppler):	Capillary refill (< 3s): ☐ Yes ☐ No	
Neck vein (distention):	Sounds: S1, S2, regular, irregular: Apical rate:	Any chest pain:

27) RESPIRATORY SYSTEM:

Depth, rate, rhythm:	Use of accessory muscles:	Cyanosis:	Sputum color, amount:	Cough: productive nonproductive	Breath sounds: clear, rales, wheezes
Use of oxygen: nasal cannula, mask, trach collar:	Flow rate of oxygen:	Oxygen humidification: ☐ Yes ☐ No		Pulse oximeter: _____ % oxygen saturation	Smoking: ☐ Yes ☐ No

28) GASTROINTESTINAL SYSTEM

Abdominal pain, tenderness, guarding; distention, soft, firm:	Bowel sounds x 4 quadrants:	NG tube: describe drainage
Ostomy: describe stoma site and stools:	Other:	

29) SKIN AND WOUNDS:

Color, turgor: **Pink**	Rash, bruises:	Describe wounds (size, locations):	Edges approximated: ☐ Yes ☐ No	Type of wound drains:
Characteristics of drainage:	Dressings (clean, dry, intact):	Sutures, staples, steri-strips, other:	Risk for pressure ulcer assessment rating:	Other:

30) EYES, EARS, NOSE, THROAT (EENT):

Eyes: redness, drainage, edema, ptosis	Ears: drainage	Nose: redness, drainage, edema	Throat: sore
Psychosocial and Cultural Assessment			
31) Religious preference (face sheet)	32) Marital status (face sheet)	33) Health care benefits and insurance (face sheet):	
34) Occupation (face sheet)	35) Emotional state (nurse's notes)		

● Figure 2.1   Patient profile database. Use blue ink for the night before clinical and a different color ink for the day of clinical. Get all of this information the night before clinical, then update it on the day of care.

Stage 2: *Autonomy Versus Shame and Doubt*

During the first few years of life, about ages 1 to 3 years, children explore their surroundings and gain increasing autonomy from their caretakers. The toddler needs much support and encouragement to learn to walk and control bowel and bladder functioning. If parents belittle the toddler, self-doubt and shame occur, and a sense of inferiority may take root.

Stage 3: *Initiative Versus Guilt*

From about ages 3 to 6 years, children begin to manipulate their environments and become very active. As they take on new challenges successfully with parental support and encouragement, children learn to take the initiative. Lack of parental support and inappropriate scolding for attempts to try new things may lead to feelings of resentment and unworthiness.

Stage 4: *Industry Versus Inferiority*

A new stage begins as the child enters school and lasts until puberty. Children must learn a new set of social rules as they enter school and develop roles and relationships with teachers and peers outside of their family. Throughout this stage, they must learn to be productive workers at school and at home. Children are expected to develop many self-care skills. They are gradually becoming independent of their families and learning about self-sufficiency. Without parental support, encouragement, and guidance, children may feel inferior and inadequate, and they may lose faith in their own ability to become self-sufficient.

Stage 5: *Ego Identity Versus Role Diffusion*

The adolescent is searching for personal identity. Establishing identity involves successful integration of many social roles, such as student, sibling, friend, cheerleader, athlete, band member, or club member. These roles must form coherent patterns that give young people a sense of who they are—their identities. Adolescents need to form close relationships with peers and to develop a sexual identity. Their value systems are evolving. They must learn to appreciate their achievements and, toward the end of this stage, select a career. Failure to accomplish this may lead to feelings of hopelessness, despair, and confusion.

Stage 6: *Intimacy Versus Isolation*

The primary task of young adulthood is to love someone else, to form an intimate bond with another person. Failure to accomplish intimacy leads to loneliness. Important tasks include maintaining friendships and establishing new social groups while taking on civic responsibilities in communities. In addition, young adults have the task of growing independent from their parents' home and managing their own households. To do so, they must establish a career. Many choose to marry. Many have their own children and take on parenting roles, which include encouraging and supporting their own children as those children attempt to accomplish the growth and developmental tasks already discussed. In addition, young adults are in the process of formulating a meaningful philosophy of life.

Stage 7: *Generativity Versus Stagnation*

During middle adulthood, the challenge is to remain productive and creative in all aspects of life and to find meaning and joy in careers, family, and community social participation. In contrast to feelings of generativity are feelings of stagnation. Life may become a boring routine, and a person may feel resentful when tasks of this stage are not successfully accomplished. To successfully accomplish this stage of life, individuals may need to review and redirect goals to achieve desired performance in a career. They also may need to develop satisfying hobby and leisure activities.

Middle adults must also accept and adjust to the physical changes of middle age, such as wearing glasses, getting wrinkles, and developing gray hair. In addition, they need to make adjustments in lifestyles to accommodate aging parents and to maintain relationships with their mates. Those with adolescent children need to assist them in searching for identity and then, as the children leave home, cope with an "empty nest" feeling. As children leave, relationships with spouses are redefined. There may be new roles of in-law and grandparent by the end of this stage.

Stage 8: *Ego Integrity Versus Despair*

During late adulthood, those with a sense of ego integrity have attained an acceptance of their lives and feelings that life has been complete and satisfactory. During this stage, individuals conduct life reviews in which they consider their successes and failures and prepare for the inevitability of death. The task is to make peace with one's self. Although the person may not have accomplished everything that she had hoped, she reconciles that it is an imperfect world, and she did the best she could, given the set of circumstances in her life. She faces death without fear, content that she has played a meaningful part in the lives of those around her. In addition, the person must continue to affiliate with others of the same age, while adjusting to the death of friends, family members, and spouse.

In contrast to ego integrity is despair. Those in despair believe that too much wrong has occurred and that there is no time to make things better. They may be filled with feelings of resentment, futility, hopelessness, and fear of death.

During this period, the tasks also include adjusting to changes in physical strength and health and arranging satisfactory physical living quarters. This includes maintaining a home or apartment or moving to a retirement center or nursing home. With retirement from the workforce, there is an adjustment to retirement and reduced income. With the loss of work roles, the person must find activities that enhance self-worth and usefulness. Some people feel free to pursue whatever activities are important to them. These activities may include a "semi-retired" career, a hobby, a sport, or community service activities.

Relevance of Growth and Development to Health State

These eight stages and their associated tasks should be foremost on your mind when you think about your patient's age. A key question is the effect a health problem and its treatment is having and will have on the person's ability to pursue the tasks of a particular age. You can assume that a person's life work has been at least temporarily altered. Depending on the health problem involved, the course of the person's life may be altered permanently. You can also assume that everyone entering a health-care setting would rather be doing their life's work and accomplishing the tasks of their age instead of working with you and the other health-care providers. The challenge to nurses is to get patients back on track and to promote optimal levels of growth and development or a peaceful death.

4) Gender

Look at the face sheet to find the patient's gender. It is important that you be aware of gender differences in communication and that you communicate clearly with both sexes. Specifically, women often are focused on affiliation through communication, wanting to establish intimacy and forming communal connections. In contrast, men tend to be focused on attaining independence and status through communication and are concerned with hierarchy in human relationships. These differing gender goals influence the nature of human relationships, including the relationships between health-care providers and patients. For example, to some men, illness may be viewed as taking away independence and status, resulting in feelings of powerlessness. But women who are functioning with affiliation goals in mind may willingly accept the support from health-care providers. As you perform assessments, be aware of gender differences in communication so that you can clearly decipher messages from both sexes.[3,4] You must look for patterns of communication in men and women, but be very mindful of stereotyping—not all women or all men will behave as described above.

5) Admission Date

Look on the face sheet for this information as well. It is important to know how long the person has been in the health-care system. With managed care, there is usually a specific amount of time allotted to each type of problem. For example, a patient having knee replacement is in the hospital for 3 to 4 days. You can begin to determine if your patient is on or off the expected course of treatment just by knowing the date of admission and the expected length of stay for the type of problem for which the patient was admitted.

6) Reason for Hospitalization

The reason for hospitalization is typed clearly on the face sheet without abbreviations. Many students struggle with abbreviations and poor handwriting, which can be avoided by obtaining the reason for hospitalization from the face sheet. This is generally a medical diagnosis and, if applicable, includes the surgical procedure. Although many things may have happened to a patient during hospitalization, it is important to know what the initial problem was that brought the person to the hospital.

7) Chronic Illnesses

The face sheet contains information on present and past chronic illnesses in addition to the reason for hospitalization. It is important to note chronic illnesses that are listed as medical diagnoses in the physician's history and progress notes. This information on chronic illness is also found on the nurse's initial intake history and physical assessment forms. These are located in the patient's chart. Many, but not all, facilities summarize pertinent information on a Kardex. The Kardex is a quick reference for nurses that contains critical information for the most current care of the patient. Facilities that use a Kardex may have slight variations in format; however, the information contained on it is almost universal.

You must look up each chronic illness and current medical diagnosis in your pathophysiology book, which will have the most complete definitions with pathological effects and the etiologies of the diseases. You should highlight all the signs and symptoms your patient exhibits at the present time. It is not at all uncommon for the same patient to have a number of chronic conditions that are different from the reason for admission. For example, a patient may have chronic diabetes and hypertension but is currently admitted for a small bowel obstruction. All medical problems must be identified and defined because you must have a clear picture of the clinical problems that may occur to develop the nursing care plan.

8) Surgical Procedures

The best place to find out what types of surgical procedures the patient underwent (or is about to undergo) is on the surgical consent forms in the patient's chart. This is because legal standards demand that the exact procedure be specified and that no abbreviations be used. The surgical procedure is also listed on the Kardex, but it may be abbreviated there and therefore more difficult to interpret.

When trying to understand the surgical procedures, you can start with a medical dictionary for a basic definition. The best reference, however, is a nursing medical-surgical text with a more detailed description of the surgical procedure. Sometimes you can find typed surgical operative notes dictated by the surgeon and transcribed by the medical records department, but these are not usually available in the chart until a few days after surgery.

9) Advance Directives

This information is found on the admission nurse's assessment form; it should also appear on the Kardex. Health-care facilities are required by law to ask patients if they have advance directives. Advance directives are legal documents, such as a living will and health-care power of attorney. A living will outlines the patient's wishes about life-sustaining treatments; typically, it tells health-care providers to withhold life-sustaining treatments if the patient is in a terminal condition and cannot make his own decisions. A health-care power of attorney appoints a person to make health-care decisions on the patient's behalf if the patient is unable to do so.

DNR is a crucial abbreviation to remember. It stands for *do not resuscitate*. If the patient has a DNR order, it will be listed on the Kardex, sometimes with a red label on the outside of the chart. It typically means that the person does not want CPR or other extreme measures performed if he goes into cardiac or respiratory arrest. The person may be given drugs and kept comfortable, and the goal is a peaceful death with dignity.

10) Laboratory Data

A specific section of the chart is set aside for the patient's laboratory values.[5] Results of the blood and urine tests described in the following sections are important to know for any patient, whether the values are normal or abnormal. Many additional tests may be ordered based on the patho-

physiology of the patient's disease. Of course, all currently abnormal results are very important because they reveal the extent of disease.

Make sure you know which tests are ordered for your clinical day of care because intravenous fluids and medication administration are directly linked to what is happening in the patient's blood and urine. You must check the new daily laboratory values before giving intravenous fluids and medications. For example, if you are giving insulin at 8 a.m., make sure you know the blood glucose value from the 6 a.m. draw. If the blood glucose value is too low, the insulin may be held. Likewise, if you are giving Lovenox (enoxaparin sodium) at 8 a.m., make sure you know results of the patient's platelet test before you give the medication. The dose of Lovenox will be held if platelet count is too low. See Table 2.1.

You should know the values of your patient's blood for the following commonly ordered blood and urine tests. These tests are universally ordered on almost all patients and serve as a baseline assessment for planning nursing care.

Inflammation and Infection:
White Blood Cells

White blood cells (WBCs), as a rule of thumb, should be fewer than 10,000/mm³. An elevation of WBCs indicates inflammation and infection. The WBCs may be subdivided into a differential count of each cell type. An increase in the number of neutrophils (band and stab cells) indicates an acute infection, also known as a "shift to the left." Other types of WBCs (basophils and eosinophils) are elevated in allergic reactions. Others (lymphocytes) are involved with developing immunity and phagocytic monocytes that

Table 2.1 Sliding Scale Insulin Dosages*	
Blood Glucose Level	Insulin Dosage
151–200 mg/dL	6 U
201–250 mg/dL	8 U
251–300 mg/dL	10 U
301–400 mg/dL	12 U

*Sample guidelines for regular sliding scale insulin. The higher the blood glucose, the more insulin is needed to regulate blood glucose levels.

engulf bacteria. A low WBC count (below 5000/mm^3) indicates problems in producing cells from the bone marrow, which may happen during chemotherapy.

Anemia and Bleeding: **Red Blood Cells, Hemoglobin, and Hematocrit**

For detecting disorders such as anemia, red blood cells (RBCs) are normally around 5.4 million/mcL for men and 4.8 million/mcL for women. Hemoglobin (Hgb) and *hematocrit* (Hct) are commonly abbreviated as H&H. Hemoglobin is a reflection of the amount of RBCs in the blood, usually 14 to 18 g/dL in male patients and 12 to 16 g/dL in female patients. The main reason that the hemoglobin level drops is bleeding. When the hemoglobin level drops below 9 g/dL, blood transfusions may be required.

Hematocrit is the percentage of RBCs in the total blood volume. The total blood volume consists of RBCs and serum. In male patients, a normal hematocrit level is 42% to 52%. In female patients, a normal hematocrit level is 37 to 47%. The hematocrit level should be about three times the Hgb concentration. When the patient is bleeding, the hematocrit level will drop along with the hemoglobin level. Hematocrit also reflects the patient's state of hydration. Sometimes the hemoglobin level is normal or slightly high, and the hematocrit level is low. This occurs when the patient is dehydrated.

Blood Coagulation Studies
These studies include platelet counts and international normalized ratio (INR), prothrombin time (PT), partial thromboplastin time (PTT), and activated partial thromboplastin time (APTT).

Platelets
Platelets are thrombocytes, which are cells essential to blood clotting. Normal platelet counts are between 150,000 to 400,000/mm^3. Platelets typically decrease because of bleeding or certain drugs hinder the bone marrow from producing these cells. For example, Lovenox (enoxaparin), which is used to prevent formation of blood clots in the legs in immobilized patients, has the side effect of decreasing platelets. For that reason, platelet counts are monitored during Lovenox

administration. The drug is usually discontinued when platelets drop below 130,000/mm^3.

INR, PT, PTT, and APTT
Values for INR, PT (sometimes called pro time), PTT, and APTT reflect different ways to express the time required for blood to coagulate and clot. The therapeutic INR level for treatment has a range of 2.0 to 3.0; PT is normally 11 to 12.5 seconds; PTT is normally 60 to 70 seconds; and APTT is normally 30 to 40 seconds. Although these values all reflect blood clotting ability, they differ somewhat: PTT or APTT is used to assess the intrinsic system of clotting, and PT or INR is used to assess the extrinsic system of clotting. These values are very important because many patients take anticoagulants to increase the time for a clot to form. For example, immobilized patients are routinely placed on anticoagulation therapy to prevent formation of blood clots. The PTT is used to assess the effects of the anticoagulant heparin, which is given subcutaneously or intravenously. The PT or INR is used to assess the effect of the anticoagulant Coumadin (warfarin), which is given orally. Heparin affects the intrinsic system of clotting, and Coumadin affects the extrinsic system of clotting.

In either case, patients receiving anticoagulant therapy will have purposely prolonged clotting times 1.5 to 2.5 times the control value. Heparin and Coumadin dosages are regulated up or down to maintain the anticoagulation at 1.5 to 2.5 times the control value. Therefore, you must know the patient's latest INR or PT before giving Coumadin, the latest APTT or PTT before giving heparin, or the latest platelet counts before giving Lovenox (enoxaparin).

Electrolytes and Cellular Functioning

One of the most important electrolytes is potassium. The normal potassium level is about 3.5 to 5.5 mEq/L. Too much or too little of this electrolyte has profound effects on all muscles, but of particular concern is the heart muscle. The ability of the heart to contract and the rate at which it contracts depend on normal potassium levels. Potassium levels typically decline with vomiting and diarrhea. Potassium-depleting diuretics are another common cause of decreased potassium levels.

Potassium is commonly added to intravenous fluids and given in oral preparations. Make sure you know the patient's latest potassium levels before giving potassium supplements, either intravenously or orally. In addition, patients taking Lanoxin (digitalis) may develop toxic levels of this drug in their bloodstream when potassium levels are too low, inducing serious cardiac arrhythmias.

There are a few other important electrolyes to monitor. For example, serum sodium (135–145 mEq/L) and chloride (97–107 mEq/L) are important in the regulation of water balance and pH. Calcium (8.2–10.2 mg/dL) and phosphorus (2.5–4.5 mg/dL) are important for bone strength and muscle functioning (including the heart muscle).

All electrolytes must be balanced carefully through appropriate oral nutrition and oral vitamin and mineral supplementations. It the patient is not able to ingest or digest the appropriate foods, then intravenous therapy will be instituted to maintain fluid and electrolyte balance.

Nutrition: **Blood Glucose, Glycosylated Hemoglobin, Cholesterol**

These tests are used to assess a patient's current glucose level and long-term glucose control.

Blood Glucose
The level of glucose in a patient's blood after fasting (also known as the fasting blood sugar) is normally 70 to 110 mg/dL of blood. Persistently elevated blood glucose levels may indicate diabetes mellitus. Because diabetes is so common, this is a common test.

Typically, when the blood glucose level is too low, the cause is unintentional insulin overdose. Consider this example: A patient's 6 a.m. glucose level is within normal limits, so the nurse gives the patient's 7 a.m. insulin, thinking that he will be eating breakfast. But the patient begins feeling nauseated and does not eat. In this case, expect an insulin reaction because the blood glucose level is guaranteed to drop.

Patients who are "brittle," which means that their blood glucose is not under control and can fluctuate widely, should be checked in the morning, usually around 6 a.m. The result of this test is the fasting blood glucose. Nonfasting blood glucose levels are commonly checked before lunch, before supper, and at bedtime. In brittle diabetics, insulin is given on a sliding scale based on the blood glucose readings.

Glycosylated Hemoglobin
Glycosylated hemoglobin (also called glycohemoglobin) is another common test of blood glucose. It is used to measure long-term blood glucose control over a period of up to 120 days. Glucose binds to hemoglobin in a chemical reaction. When the patient is diabetic and blood glucose levels are elevated, the percentage of glycosylated hemoglobin is higher. This reaction is not reversible; once the glycogen attaches, it remains with RBC for its life cycle, about 120 days. Therefore, you can tell if the patient's blood glucose has been under control over time. Normal, healthy people have 5.5% to 8.8% of total hemoglobin bound to glucose. Diabetics under control range from 7.5% to 11.4% total hemoglobin bound to glucose, whereas those who need either more diet instruction or more insulin (or both) will be higher. There are three types of hemoglobin that become glycosylated: A1a, A1b, and A1c. Many laboratories report only the A1c level, which is normally 3.56% bound to glucose.[6]

Cholesterol. The cholesterol level indicates the amount of lipids or fats in the blood. Lipids are carried in the blood in combination with proteins and are thus called lipoproteins. High levels of cholesterol are a risk factor for cardiovascular disease, which is the primary health problem in the United States. Numerous people have cholesterol levels above 200 mg/dL. Cholesterol is composed of high-density lipoproteins (HDL), low-density lipoproteins (LDLs), and triglycerides.

Of primary interest in relation to cardiac disease are the LDLs, which should be less than 130 mg/dL. LDLs have been called "bad" cholesterol because they produce atherosclerosis. Many people take lipid-lowering drugs such as Lipitor (atorvastatin calcium) to reduce their LDL levels. They also are prescribed a low cholesterol diet and exercise program.

Kidney Functioning. Blood urea nitrogen and creatinine levels are commonly used to determine the functioning of the kidneys. Normally, creatinine values are <1.5 mg/dL, and blood urea nitrogen ranges from 8 to 23 mg/dL.

Urine analysis is done mainly to check for infection and also to check kidney function. Bladder infections are extremely common, especially in women because they have a shorter urethra than men. Typically, a clean catch urine specimen is obtained. The patient wipes the urethra with special antiseptic solution, voids a little in the toilet, and then inserts a sterile cup under the urine stream until the cup contains about 30 mL. This specimen should contain fewer than 10,000 bacteria/mL, provided the patient has wiped the urethra properly to decrease the number of normal flora around the meatus. A specimen obtained from a sterile catheterization, where a sterile tube is inserted into the sterile bladder, should contain no bacteria. In addition, the urine should contain no protein, blood, ketones, or glucose. Any of these substances in urine usually indicate diabetes or kidney disease.

Liver Functioning. Bilirubin is the product of the breakdown of RBCs by the liver. Normal values are 0.3 to 1.1 mg/dL. With liver failure, the bilirubin levels rise, and the patient becomes jaundiced. There are three important liver enzymes: Alkaline phosphatase (ALP), normally 35 to 142 U/L in males and 25 to 125 U/L in females; aspartate aminotransferase (AST), normally 19 to 48 U/L in males and 9 to 36 U/L in females; and alanine aminotransferase (ALT), normally 10 to 40 U/L in males and 7 to 35 U/L in females. These values will all be elevated with liver disease, such as hepatitis, cirrhosis, and liver failure. A functioning liver is crucial to the metabolism of drugs, and many drugs can damage the liver, so monitoring the functioning of the liver is very important.

Heart Functioning. Blood studies analyze functioning of the heart. For example, tests for diagnosis of myocardial infarction include blood levels of creatine kinase (CK), normally 38 to 174 U/L in males and 26 to 140 U/L in females. CK-MB, specific to myocardial cells, is normally less than 4% to 6% of the total CK values. Elevations in CK indicate damage to myocardial cells during acute myocardial infarction, when CK is released into the serum from damaged myocardial cells within the first 48 hours, and CK-MBs appear in the first 6 to 24 hours. With heart muscle damage, troponin 1 (normally <0.35 ng/mL) and troponin T (normally < 0.20 mcg/L) will be elevated between 2 and 6 hours following myocardial infarction. In addition, B-natriuretic peptide (BNP) (normally <100 pg/mL) serum values increase in proportion to the extent of congestive heart failure. BNP is produced in the left ventricle with increased ventricular pressure and volume of blood in the ventricle, which are the result of heart failure.

Respirator Functioning and Acid Base Balance. Blood gases are analyzed whenever respiratory functioning is of concern and the patient may not be getting enough oxygen. An arterial blood sample is obtained to determine the amount of oxygen in the blood (pO_2); it is normally 80 to 95 mm Hg and will be decreased without adequate respirations. In addition, carbon dioxide levels (pCO_2), normally 35 to 45 mm Hg, will rise without adequate respirations. As the patient lacks oxygen and becomes hypoxic, he becomes acidic, and the pH (normally 7.35–7.45) will decrease. In addition, bicarbonate (HCO_3), (normally 18–23 mEq/L) is also measured. In response to respiratory acidosis, the kidneys will retain the base bicarbonate to compensate for the acidosis (which was due to respiratory failure), and bicarbonate levels will rise.

Always record any recent abnormal values (within 1 day of your clinical assignment), and record what the values were on admission. Laboratory reports are very important in determining the extent of the patient's chronic and acute diseases and the outcomes of surgery, such as the amount of blood loss during surgery, or if the patient continues to bleed following surgery. Medication administration and medical treatments are based on the results of laboratory reports. The goal will be to develop a care map that reflects the coordination of pathology and assessment data with laboratory data and medications and treatments used to control chronic and acute responses to health problems.

11) Diagnostic Tests

Your patient may undergo a wide range of diagnostic tests. Perhaps the two most common tests are a chest x-ray and an electrocardiogram (EKG).

Chest X-Ray

You can find chest x-ray reports in the patient's chart under laboratory and diagnostic procedures. The chest x-ray is a basic diagnostic test used to examine the structure of the heart and lungs. Enlargement of the heart and areas of lung consolidation, which could result from pneumonia or tumors, can be detected on chest x-rays.

EKG

The EKG indicates patterns of electrical activity and contraction of the heart muscle. This test is routinely obtained on patients over age 35 as part of a general physical examination. This report is also found under laboratory and diagnostic procedures in the patient's chart. Although student nurses are not expected to interpret EKG tracings, the interpretation is printed on the report along with the rhythm strips indicating the rate and rhythm of the heart.

Sputum and Blood Cultures

Sputum specimens coughed up from the lungs are used to determine the type of microorganism that is causing an infection of the lungs. Blood cultures are obtained when the patient is believed to be septic and an infecting organism has been spread systemically throughout the body. Sputum or blood specimens are smeared on a culture plate and incubated to grow the bacteria. Then bacteria are examined under a microscope, and the types of drugs that may be used to kill the organism are determined.

12) Medications

One of the most important, and dangerous, tasks for which nurses are responsible is medication administration. Include all drugs the patient is taking that are prescriptions written by physicians as well as over the counter (OTC) and herbal medications taken by the patient. Alternative therapy OTC preparations and herbal remedies have become very important in treatment regimes. From virtually the first day of classes, nurses learn the six "rights" of drug administration:

- Right drug
- Right patient
- Right dose
- Right route
- Right time
- Right to refuse a medication

This sounds simple enough; yet, despite the best intentions of nurses and other health-care professionals, medication errors occur. They can harm or kill patients. Consequently, you must be exceedingly careful whenever you work with medications.

To find information about your patient's medications, look on the medication sheet, also known as the medication record, which is usually kept in the same place as the Kardex. List each drug and the times it should be administered on your patient profile database. Sometimes, drugs are misspelled on these sheets. Therefore, you should go directly to the patients' medication drawer or wherever drugs are kept and copy the name and dosage of the drug from the paper wrapper on the drug. That way, you can be sure you have spelled the drug name correctly.

When you get home, you will need to look up and study each drug. You may want to consider purchasing a drug book or set of drug cards so you can highlight important actions and side effects on the cards. Computer programs are also available for drug information, and they save time in finding information. Also consider looking on the Internet for drug information. Keep in mind that not every drug is available in any given drug reference. Be very careful that you have a valid and reliable source of information when obtaining information from the Internet.

If you are unable to find a drug in your reference book or computer program, call the pharmacy at the health-care institution or the pharmacist at the local drug store. Tell the pharmacist that you are a nursing student and would like information on a drug. For example, suppose you cannot find Alu-Tab tablets in your drug cards. Ask the pharmacist to give you information about that drug over the phone.

As you research your drugs, always write down the times the drug is to be administered, the brand/trade name, and the generic name of the drug. Many times the brand/trade name is listed on a medication record, but a generic drug is substituted by the pharmacy. Sometimes, two generic drugs will be substituted for a single combination trade-name drug. This may be confusing at first. For example, the trade-name drug Diovan HCT contains both valsartan and hydrochlorothiazide in one tablet. The pharmacy may substitute two generic tablets: one tablet of valsartan and one tablet of hydrochlorothiazide. Substitutes are made by pharmacies to decrease the cost of brand-name drugs. You must know the composition of each tablet to be administered, and you must be especially careful when combination drugs have been ordered.

You should know the dose to be administered and if the dose is within the recommended range of the manufacturer of the drug. Identify how the drug is to be administered, also known as the route of administration. Be sure that the dose of the drug is compatible with the route of administration.

It is most important to recognize the general classification to which any particular drug belongs. This will help you in identifying where the drug belongs on the care map. For example:

- Antibiotics are grouped with the nursing diagnosis related to the area of a problem, such as *Impaired Urinary Elimination* if the patient has a urinary tract infection.
- Antidysrhythmics and antihypertensives are grouped with *Decreased Cardiac Output*
- Anticoagulants and diuretics are grouped with *Deficient Fluid Volume*
- Corticosteroids are grouped with *Ineffective Protection*
- Anticonvulsants are grouped with *Ineffective Tissue Perfusion (cerebral)*
- Insulins are grouped with *Imbalanced Nutrition: less than body requirements*
- Drugs used for pain are grouped with *Acute Pain* or *Chronic Pain*

For each drug, you must determine the actions of the drug. Many times there is more than one action of a drug. Then, identify the specific reason your patient is receiving the drug. For example, determine if your patient is taking aspirin for pain, to reduce a temperature, or as a blood thinner.

You must be aware of the pharmacokinetics of each drug. Specifically, understand the onset (O), peak (P), duration (D), and half-life ($1/2$) of the drug. In addition, find out how the drug is metabolized (M) and excreted (E) from the body. Many drugs are metabolized in the liver and excreted by the kidneys. Therefore you must know the status of liver and renal functioning through analysis of laboratory data as described in the section on collection of laboratory data.

Contraindications for the drugs are also important. Under what conditions should the patient not take the drug? What are the major adverse effects or side effects of each drug? Every drug has side effects, which must be carefully monitored in patients. For example, the side effects of many antibiotics include nausea and diarrhea.

Nursing implications include what the nurse should assess while the patient is taking the drug. If a patient is on a blood pressure medication, the nurse should know what the patient's blood pressure is prior to administration of the drug. If the nurse is administering potassium, the nurse should know the potassium level. In addition, there is patient/family teaching to be done with each drug. The patient must be taught everything he needs to know to take care of himself at home if he is to be discharged with the drug and at least the purpose of the drug to be administered while hospitalized.

13) Allergies

Allergies to drugs may appear in many places in patient records. Allergies to drugs are critical to note because an allergic reaction may lead to anaphylactic shock and death. In many institutions, the front of the chart will have a red label on it noting drug allergies. The medication record will have a space for drug allergies, and the Kardex will also list drug allergies.

14) Pain Medications and Pain Ratings

Pain control is a task central to nursing care. Find out when the patient last received a pain medication, what type of medication it was, and the amount administered. You can find this information on the medication administration record. Look at the pattern of pain medication administration. This will give you an indication of the amount of pain the patient has been having. However, keep in mind that not all patients will ask for pain medication, even when they are uncomfortable.

Pain Ratings

A patient's perception of pain is documented on the flow sheets and on the nurses' notes. Patients are usually asked to rate the amount of pain they feel on a scale of 0 to 10, with 0 as no pain and 10 as the worst pain ever experienced. You need to locate the most recent pain rating on the nursing notes. Subjective pain ratings can be used in addition to the data collected about the patient's use of pain medications. In addition, the nurses' notes will also indicate the location of the patient's pain.

15) Treatments and Relation to Medical and Nursing Diagnoses

Examples of patient treatments include oxygen administration, incentive spirometry, catheters, nasogastric tubes, and dressing changes. You will eventually be responsible for ensuring that all treatments are done. The treatments are listed on the Kardex. It is important to note what these treatments are, even if you have not yet learned how to perform them. Your agency nurse may actually perform a treatment that you have not yet learned how to do.

You must know the rationale for each of the treatments. Look up and define each treatment, and know why the patient is receiving the treatment as it relates to the medical and nursing diagnoses. For example, the patient may be instructed to do incentive spirometry breathing exercises every hour while awake to promote deep breathing and oxygenation in the lungs and to prevent pneumonia. When you make your map of major nursing diagnoses, this treatment will be grouped under the nursing diagnosis of *Impaired Gas Exchange.*

16) Support Services

Support services represent all the disciplines involved in the patient's care. These include nutrition, physical, occupational, speech, and respiratory therapy and social work. It is important to identify the role of each discipline in the patient's care. The nurse's role is to assess the patient's health state and to recognize whether the patient will be able to tolerate the services that are scheduled. The nurse then communicates as appropriate with the support services

and the attending physician and gives recommendations for therapy.

For example, a patient is supposed to be ambulated in the hall after a total hip replacement. You know that the patient's morning hemoglobin was 8 g/dL, the patient is scheduled for a transfusion, her blood pressure was lower than it was yesterday, her face is pale, and her nailbeds are white. You are responsible for discussing patient data with the physical therapist and recommending that the patient be exercised in bed and ambulated to a chair and that the physical therapist should wait until after the transfusion to get the patient up and walking in the hall.

In another example, a patient has asthma and receives inhalation treatments every 4 hours. You note that the patient's breathing is worsening even though the 4 hours have not elapsed. You should intervene and call the respiratory therapist to report the problem and ask if the therapist could arrive right on time or even a few minutes early for the next treatment.

17) Consultations

Consultants are physicians who are specialists, such as cardiologists, pulmonologists, and gastroenterologists. They are listed on the Kardex in the patient's chart. The primary doctor who admitted the patient to the hospital will call in a specialist when he or she suspects that the patient's medical problem resides in a specific organ system. In essence, the primary doctor is asking the opinion and treatment advice of the specialist. If you know the specialty of the consultants, you know which physiological components of the body to assess most carefully, because the primary physician would not need the services of the consultant unless something was likely to be wrong with that system of the body. Consultants typically focus on one body system.

18) Type of Diet

The type of diet the patient is following and any dietary restrictions are always listed on the Kardex. The nursing diagnosis *Imbalanced Nutrition* is very common, and patients often have knowledge deficits and problems in managing and adhering to prescribed diets. A regular or general diet is based on the food pyramid guidelines issued by the U.S. government, which is shown in Figure 2.2. The most common types of special and restricted diets are described below.

NPO

Many patients are NPO *(nulla/nil/non per os)* (Latin for nothing by mouth) for surgery or for diagnostic testing to prevent aspiration during procedures.

Liquid Diet

After surgery or tests for which the patient has been NPO, he may receive clear liquids because they are easy to digest. Also, surgical patients who may be nauseated by anesthesia and pain medications tolerate clear liquids best. The clear liquid diet is missing many nutrients, but it does provide fluids.

Clear liquids include anything that you can see through, such as tea, 7-Up, apple juice, Sprite, ginger ale, Popsicles, Jello, sherbet, and broth. Orange juice and coffee, two of the most common drinks, should be avoided in nauseated patients because they are acidic and likely to induce vomiting. As nausea improves, the patient can be advanced to full liquids, which include milk, ice cream, fruit juices, and cooked cereals.

Soft Diet

A soft diet is commonly prescribed for stroke patients, patients without teeth, and patients who have had throat surgery—in short, for anyone who has trouble chewing or swallowing. Stroke patients have trouble chewing and swallowing because of paralysis. After throat surgery, patients may have problems swallowing because of pain. To make a soft diet, regular foods from the food pyramid can be put into a food processor and pureed. Patients at home may opt to buy strained baby food from the grocery store.

Low-Fat Diet

A low-fat diet may be recommended for patients with cardiovascular disease, hypertension, or gallbladder disease. In cardiovascular disease, low-fat diets are recommended to decrease high cholesterol levels. Low-fat diets are also used to control gallbladder spasm with gallbladder disease, as fat in the intestines prompts the gallbladder to release bile to digest the fat. If the gallbladder ducts are obstructed by stones or other pathology, spasms can be very painful and cause what is commonly called a gallbladder "attack."

Low-Sodium Diet

Patients with cardiovascular disease are commonly put on low-sodium diets to reduce fluid retention, because anywhere sodium goes water always follows. Cardiac patients commonly retain fluids, so limited amounts of sodium are allowed in the diet to promote excretion of extra fluids. Sometimes cardiac patients are also placed on fluid restrictions.

Low-Protein Diet

Low-protein diets are common among patients with liver and kidney failure. The liver normally metabolizes protein breakdown products, such as nitrogenous ammonia. Without conversion of ammonia to urea for excretion by the kidneys, ammonia levels build in the blood. Ammonia crosses the blood-brain barrier and results in encephalopathy (malfunction of the brain), in which the patient will have symptoms such as disorientation, decreased levels of consciousness, and sensory deficits.

In renal failure, low-protein diets are also common because the kidneys are unable to excrete urea. Although the liver functions and produces urea, the kidneys can no longer excrete urea. Thus, levels of blood urea nitrogen (BUN) increase, urea crosses the blood-brain barrier, and encephalopathy results.

Low-Sugar Diet

Diabetic patients are unable to break down sugar (glucose) for use by any cells of the body. That means diabetics can eat very little candy, cake, pie, or other foods that contain high concentrations of sugar. Diabetes is treated by controlling the total number of calories along with the portions of protein, fat, and carbohydrates in all food taken into the body.

Food intake must be regulated in conjunction with the quantity of insulin given as well as the amount of daily exercise activities. Diabetics must learn to eat balanced meals and snacks that contain healthy foods low in sugar and cholesterol. Food exchange lists are based on the food pyramid shown in Figure 2.2. These lists show what counts as a serving of meat, fruit, milk, vegetables, or fat. For a sample daily menu, the patient may be told to eat:

▶ 1 fruit, 2 breads, 1 milk, and 1 tsp fat for breakfast
▶ 2 oz of meat, 3 breads, 1 tsp fat, 1 vegetable, and 1 fruit for lunch
▶ 3 oz of meat, 2 breads, 2 tsp fat, and 2 vegetables for supper
▶ A snack of 1 milk, 1 bread, and 1 tsp fat

Weight Reduction Diet

Weight reduction diets control calories while providing all the nutrients essential for health. Healthy weight reduction diets use food exchange lists in a manner very similar to diabetic diets, balancing fruits, breads, vegetables, meats, and fats consumed during each meal. Weight reduction diets should not go below 1200 calories a day because it is nearly impossible to obtain the essential nutrients needed each day in fewer than 1200 calories.

Food is fuel for the body. Every activity requires fuel to produce energy. To lose weight, the patient must burn more calories than are consumed. Loss of 1 pound in a week will require burning 3500 calories through dieting.

Exercise is an important component of any weight reduction plan. The patient will increase the amount of energy used by burning more calories through exercise, thus improving weight loss. Added benefits from exercise include improved muscle tone and overall stamina. A health goal is to gradually build up to walking a minimum of 30 minutes a day, at least 4 days a week.

High-Fiber Diet

High-fiber diets are typically recommended to promote healthy bowel functioning and normal bowel movements. High-fiber foods include whole grain or bran breads and cereals or food with skins or seeds.

Low-Residue Diet

Patients with inflammatory bowel disease such as colitis, enteritis, or Crohn's disease commonly cannot tolerate foods high in fiber. These patients are placed on low-residue diets. Residue refers to the indigestible substances left in the gastrointestinal tract after digestion and absorption have occurred. With inflammation of the bowel, fibrous foods can be irritating and cause pain. Low-residue foods are mild in flavor, well cooked, and tender. Tender cuts of meat, canned fruits, cottage cheese, and white low-fiber breads are examples of foods in this diet.

Bland Diet

Sometimes, patients with gastrointestinal or bowel problems may be placed on bland diets, which are chemically and mechanically nonstimulating. Thus, these diets include bland and soft foods.

Tube Feeding

If the patient can digest food but cannot chew or swallow, he may receive food through a tube threaded into his stomach. This is called tube feeding. The tube may be passed from the nose to the stomach (nasogastric [NG] tube), or it may be surgically inserted through the abdominal wall into the stomach (gastric tube [G-tube]).

A liquid food formula that contains all nutrients needed to maintain health is infused down the tube directly to the patient's stomach, bypassing the throat to avoid aspiration. The patient may have a continuous feeding, with a machine continually pumping formula at a specific hourly rate, or the patient may receive bolus feedings, in which a specific amount of formula is given all at one time. The patient typically receives a bolus at breakfast, lunch, dinner, and bedtime.

The type or brand of tube feeding, the amount to be infused in milliliters per hour, or the amount to be given in a bolus will appear in the Kardex under diet. Also, go to the patient's room or the kitchen, and look at the cans of formula. Record the amount of protein, fat, and carbohydrate in each can. There are many types of food formulas designed to meet patients' special dietary needs. For example, special tube feeding formulas have been manufactured to contain reduced protein or partially digested protein for patients who have renal failure or liver failure.

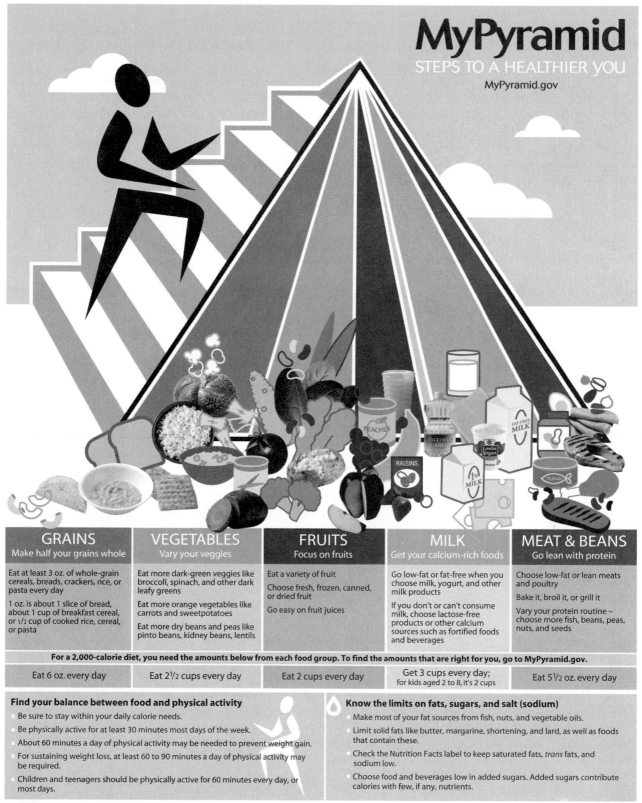

● Figure 2.2   Nutrition pyramid.

Priority Nutrition Assessments

Patients who are confused or paralyzed or who have decreased levels of consciousness, regardless of disorder, will need assistance and monitoring to maintain a diet successfully. These patients have trouble putting food to their mouths, chewing food, or swallowing food. If a patient cannot chew or swallow, he may choke and aspirate food into his lungs. For example, a patient who has had a stroke may be paralyzed on one side of his mouth and throat and may have decreased levels of consciousness.

Perform a careful assessment of the patient who has had his throat numbed because he will be temporarily unable to swallow. For example, following a bronchoscopy or endoscopy procedure, the gag reflex is temporarily paralyzed to facilitate passage of the tube into the lungs, stomach, or small intestine. Never feed someone after such a procedure until you check for a gag reflex, and make sure it has returned. As you consider the patient's diagnosis and procedures, always consider the effect on the patient's ability to move his arms and place food into his own mouth as well as his ability to swallow and chew.

The patient's appetite and amount of food consumed is usually listed as a specific percentage of food eaten off a tray, such as 50% of breakfast, 25% of lunch, or 100% of supper. The amount of food consumed is generally found in the nurses' notes or on the nursing flow sheets. Flow sheets are a special form of nurses' notes used to record routine observations such as diet. In addition, any record of problems with nausea, vomiting, or diarrhea will be found in the nurses' notes.

Many patients have problems with fluid balance and need to have their fluid intake and urinary output monitored to track the milliliters of fluid taken in and the amount of urine and other drainages during each shift. Fluid intake and output for each shift is added together to compute the fluid intake and output for 24 hours. Fluid intake and output is recorded on the nursing intake and output flow sheets. Fluid intake should approximately equal fluid output in a healthy state. If a patient is overhydrated and retains fluids, she may exhibit edema. In that case, intake has exceeded output. In contrast, if the patient is dehydrated, she has lost fluids, and output has exceeded intake.

19) Intravenous Fluids

Fluids may also be given intravenously to replace fluids and electrolytes or to feed patients when gastrointestinal pathology prevents adequate absorption of water or nutrients. Intravenous (IV) lines are also used to administer drugs. A small tube or catheter is inserted directly into a vein, leading from the vein to a bag of fluids. The solution flows out of the bag, through the tube, and into the vein. Nurses may regulate flow rates for IV lines manually by opening or closing a small clamp on the tubing. In many cases, the flow is controlled by an electric pump.

The type and rate of fluid for administration will be found on the Kardex. A special IV therapy record is also kept to document the entire course of IV solutions the patient has received. This record is similar to the medication record. Even if you have not yet learned how to manage an IV, it is important to note on your database that the patient has an IV line because this is the first step in relating this treatment to the underlying pathology. The presence of an IV means that the patient cannot take fluids, electrolytes, nutrients, or medications orally; otherwise, the IV line would be discontinued.

There are many types of IV fluids used, such as dextrose 5% in water (D_5W), lactated Ringer's (LR) solution, and normal saline (NS) solution. If you do not recognize the abbreviations used in a patient's chart, one way to find out exactly what is in the bag is to look at the bag as it hangs near the patient. Once you find out what is in the bag, you can figure out how IV therapy is related to the medical and nursing diagnoses. For example, a dehydrated patient has a fluid volume deficit; therefore she is receiving dextrose and water to replace fluids.

An IV line is a potential source of infection because a catheter is going directly into the bloodstream. Therefore, nurses look carefully at where the needle is inserted under the skin and record any signs and symptoms of inflammation, such as redness, swelling, or pain at the site. The dressing over the site must be dry and intact. All of this will be noted on the IV therapy record. The total amount of IV fluids given for the day is also recorded on the nursing flow sheets under intake for the shift.

20) Elimination

Nurses keep track of elimination very carefully. What goes in has to come out on a regular basis, or else the patient will develop a problem. Elimination includes urine output and bowel movements.

The amount of urine in milliliters appears on the flow sheet. Any abnormalities in urine color, odor, and quantity is recorded in the nurses' shift assessment notes, along with pain on elimination or incontinence (loss of control over the bladder with involuntary urination).

Knowing the patient's urine output is very important. For example, decreased urine output could cause or worsen problems of heart failure. Decreased urine output could also indicate renal failure. As you study the pathophysiology of disease, you will recognize how fluid volume deficits and excesses are manifestations of diseases that need to be carefully tracked. Something must be done to treat the patient if the urine output is too high or too low.

Many patients have a special tube to drain urine called a urinary catheter. The tube is usually held in place in the bladder with a balloon. In male patients, it may be held in place externally with a condom-like attachment. The tube leads to a drainage bag. Any patient who has a catheter has an elimination problem, or the tube would not be needed. You need to consider why the catheter is needed as it relates to the medical and nursing diagnoses. For example, a catheter may be needed in almost anyone with surgery of the genitourinary system; watch for bleeding in the urine, and keep track of the output.

Bowel movements are also very important because any patient who is immobilized for any reason may be prone to constipation due to decreased peristalsis. Therefore, bowel movements are monitored and recorded on the flow sheets, and any abnormality is documented in the nurses' shift assessment notes. Check the flow sheet to determine when the patient last had a bowel movement, and check the nurses' notes about problems with constipation, diarrhea, flatus, emesis, or involuntary bowel movements.

Constipation can lead to abdominal discomfort and even impaction, in which the stool creates a blockage and obstructs the bowel. If the bowel is not functioning, the patient may have problems with belching (eructation) or vomiting (emesis). If gas and solid wastes cannot pass downward and out of the rectum, they will come out the other end of the gastrointestinal tract as evidenced by belching and emesis.

Postoperatively, patients typically have a decline in bowel functioning because they have been without regular meals. This decline is also due to the decrease in peristalsis that results from immobility and the adverse effects of anesthesia and narcotic pain medications. A healthy sign is the passing of flatus (gas) from the anus. Even though patients have not yet had a bowel movement, a bowel movement may be impending.

21) Activity

The Kardex will list the patient's activity orders. It is crucial to know what the patient can and cannot do regarding activities to keep her safe from injuries. Carefully assess the patient's ability to walk. The patient's gait may be documented as steady or nonsteady. Note the use of assistive devices such as canes, walkers, or prostheses. The patient may be ordered to bedrest, chair, bathroom privileges (BRP), up as tolerated, and so on at the physician's discretion. In hospital settings, patients who are confused or have a decreased level of consciousness may need restraints or all side rails up on the bed.

In orthopedic patients, knowing the percentage of weightbearing on the injured bone is essential to prevent falls or further injury to the bone. Typically, weightbearing is described as a percentage, such as 25% on the right knee, 50% on the left hip, or toe-touch only. Abbreviations may be used for terms such as no weightbearing (NWB) or weightbearing as tolerated (WBAT).

A major concern with activity is that the patient does not fall. Preventing patient falls is a primary safety issue. Each patient has a fall risk assessment done routinely. This fall assessment is required by JCAHO and is a very specific standard of care. Examples of patients who are at high risk for falls include those with decreased levels of consciousness, those with sensory deficits, those receiving pain medications, and those receiving antihypertensive drugs. Review your patient's fall assessment profile, and update it to the best of your knowledge based on the data collected. If the risk for falls is great, restraints may be used for safety.

Sleeping is a very important activity. The nurses' notes will indicate whether the patient had any problems sleeping. Sleep is an important restorative function and promotes physical healing and cognitive function. Sleep deprivation has many negative consequences, including irritability and increased sensitivity to pain.

Routine Physical Assessment

In inpatient and outpatient settings, routine head-to-toe physical assessment information is gathered at the beginning of the shift or on entry into the outpatient setting. You need to find the most recent physical assessment data available for the patient. Most agencies use a standardized assessment form that contains a checklist with some space for comments. Nurses expand on problem areas in the nurses' notes. When a system to be assessed is within acceptable limits, the nurse may need to document by writing only *within normal limits* (WNL) or *within designated limits* (WDL). Not writing about normal findings saves much time and is called charting by exception. Documentation is explained in more detail in Chapter 7.

Nurses are required to perform at least one full assessment per shift and check any abnormalities in the assessment much more frequently. As you complete your database patient profile, always record the latest physical assessment data by checking the most recent physical assessment information. The following head-to-toe assessment serves as a review of important information to note on the patient profile database.

22) Vital Signs

Vital signs include blood pressure (BP), temperature (T), pulse (P), and respirations (R). These data provide "vital" information about the key organ systems of the body. The cardiovascular system is assessed by blood pressure and pulse, whereas the lungs are assessed by respirations. Immune functioning, specifically infection, is assessed by body temperature. The patient's most recent vital signs may be located on a tempera-

ture clipboard because they are often collected by ancillary personnel who may not write directly on the flow sheets.

23) Height and Weight

Height and weight give an indication of the patient's basic nutritional status. This is found in the nursing admission assessment information.

Review of Systems

In a review of systems, which is the major portion of the physical assessment, each system of the body is assessed using the techniques of inspection, palpation, percussion, and auscultation. This information is vital to developing basic nursing diagnoses. Pay close attention to what has been recorded in the most recent nursing notes and nursing assessments.

24) Neurological and Mental Status

The functioning of the brain is assessed by determining the level of consciousness (LOC) and whether the patient is alert and oriented to person, place, and time of day or if he is confused or disoriented. The patient's speech should be clear and appropriate. The patient's pupils must be equal, round, and reactive to light and accommodation (PERRLA). In addition, the patient should have no deficits in the senses of hearing, vision, taste, or smell. Deficits in any of these areas place the person at high risk for injury as a primary diagnosis. Other nursing diagnoses may include *Self-care Deficit, Disturbed Sensory Perception, Impaired Verbal Communication, Acute or Chronic Confusion,* and *Impaired Memory.* The brain controls all motor movements of the body. Motor status is assessed by the patient's ability to move both arms and both legs and to feel sensation, such as pressure and pain, in all limbs. Motor status is recorded with the musculoskeletal system on the patient profile database.

25) Musculoskeletal Status

Musculoskeletal problems are classified under the nursing diagnoses *Activity Intolerance* and *Impaired Physical Mobility.* Deficits in bones, muscles, and joints usually occupy one of the following categories:

▶ Fracture—any type of break or crack in a bone
▶ Contracture—tightening and shrinking of the muscles from paralysis or fibrosis
▶ Arthritis—inflammation of a joint
▶ Spinal curvature—deformed twisting of the bones of the spine

The range of motion (ROM) of each extremity must be recorded under motor abilities. Full ROM is normal, with decreased ROM and strength as a result of pathology. Circulation is another important aspect of the musculoskeletal database. A circulation check is an assessment of blood flow to the extremities. Most important, circulation checks include the distal pulses, such as the pedal and tibial pulses in the feet and the radial pulse in the wrist. During the assessment, the nurse observes for pallor, warmth, or coolness of the skin; the patient's sense of touch on the injured limb; the amount of edema or swelling in the limb; and the amount of pain reported.

Pulse is the most important information about circulation to the limbs. If a pulse is not palpable, a Doppler machine is used to amplify the sound of the pulse in the artery. Lack of a pulse in a limb is a medical emergency. It means that there is no blood circulating to the limb; the tissues will die without oxygen. If the situation is not immediately rectified, it may result in the need to amputate the limb. Pulses in the extremities also indicate the ability of the heart to effectively pump blood to the periphery of the body.

When bones are broken, the patient may need a cast, splint, brace, collar, or other device to immobilize muscles, tendons, or bones. Anyone in a cast needs circulation checks. Sometimes, edema causes a cast to become too tight, cutting off circulation in the limb. The cast will need to be removed to restore circulation or else risk tissue death and the need for amputation of the affected extremity.

Therapeutic treatment devices are often required to improve circulation in the limbs. Circulation decreases when the patient is immobilized. With immobility, blood stagnates in the limbs, raising the risk of serious complications such as thrombus formation, thrombophlebitis, and embolism. A thrombus is a blood clot in the leg veins that irritates and inflames the vessel (thrombophlebitis). If the thrombus breaks off and floats freely in the bloodstream, it is called an embolus and can subsequently lodge in a blood vessel in the lung (pulmonary embolism). The reason for treating patients with antiembolic stockings, mechanical plexi pulses, or sequential compression devices is to improve venous circulation and return to the heart, thereby preventing thrombus formation.

26) Cardiovascular System

The basic assessment of the heart includes listening to heart sounds and determining if the sounds are normal or abnormal, determining if the heart is beating regularly or irregularly, and assessing for chest pain. The apical pulse rate is assessed at the apical area of the heart, but a thorough assessment includes listening in the aortic, pulmonic, tricuspid, and mitral areas as well. Abnormal heart sounds and rates appear under the nursing diagnosis *Decreased Cardiac Output*. An indication of congestive heart failure, in which the heart no longer pumps fluids effectively, is engorgement of the neck veins. Engorged neck veins are referred to as jugular venous distention (JVD). Chest pain, also known as angina, is a very important symptom that indicates the heart is not getting enough oxygen. Chest pain needs to be treated immediately, especially in a patient with a chronic or acute condition involving the cardiac system.

Assessment of the peripheral vascular system includes assessing all pulses, the same as for musculoskeletal assessment. Pulses in the limbs are especially important to check because doing so helps you assess the heart's ability to pump blood to the extremities. If the pulses are not palpable, using the Doppler device to hear them is the appropriate procedure to check adequate circulation in the limb.

The color of the nailbeds and capillary refill in the nails are also indications of circulation. The nailbeds should be pink. After depressing a nailbed, which evacuates the blood and turns the nail white, the pink color should return within 3 seconds after you stop depressing. The is called capillary refill time.

Edema indicates that a patient is retaining fluid because the failing heart is not able to pump the fluids efficiently, so some of the fluid filters into the surrounding tissues. Pitting edema means that when the examiner compresses the edematous area with his thumb over a bone, a dent remains in the tissue for a period, which indicates excessive fluid volume in the tissue.

27) Respiratory System

The depth, rate, rhythm, and use of accessory muscles should be carefully observed and the breath sounds auscultated for abnormalities. Breath sounds are normally clear, without crackles (rales) or wheezes. Cyanosis, a blue discoloration of the skin or nailbeds, indicates a lack of oxygen. A cough may be characterized as productive (producing sputum) or nonproductive (without sputum). When sputum is present, the color and amount is also recorded.

Oxygen therapy is commonly given to treat insufficient oxygenation, and the type of therapy is listed on the Kardex or record. Oxygen is commonly given via a nasal cannula (in which small tubes extend into the patient's nostrils), a face mask, or a tracheotomy collar. Because oxygen is quite drying to mucous membranes, it often is humidified. Note the flow rate if the patient has oxygen running.

A pulse oximeter is commonly used to evaluate oxygen saturation of hemoglobin. Record the percentage of oxygen saturation. Note whether the patient has a history of smoking. Nursing diagnoses commonly used for problems in this area include *Impaired Gas Exchange* and *Ineffective Airway Clearance.*

28) Gastrointestinal System

Bowel sounds must be present in all four quadrants of the patient's abdomen. They represent peristalsis, defined as the movement of materials through the gastrointestinal (GI) tract. Bowel sounds in all four quadrants indicate a functional GI tract. Absent or decreased bowel sounds may produce a firm and distended abdomen from the accumulation of solid waste and gas. The patient may report abdominal pain and tenderness. Decreased peristalsis may result in nausea and vomiting.

A common treatment for patients with little or no peristalsis is an NG tube. This tube is inserted into the stomach and attached to suction to remove solids, fluids, and gases until bowel functioning returns to normal. Drainage is carefully measured as part of the patient's output. The color of the output is also described. For example: brown, black, or "coffee ground" drainage may be caused by old dried blood, whereas green indicates bile in the drainage.

Some patients may have an ostomy, which is a surgical opening across the abdominal wall. The intestine is cut and sewn onto the opening. If the ostomy involves the colon, the opening is called a colostomy. If it involves the ileum portion of the intestine, it is called an ileostomy. A plastic bag is glued to the abdomen to catch the wastes that would normally be evacuated from the rectum. This surgical procedure is usually done to treat cancer of the bowel, when the cancerous portion of the bowel is removed. The color, consistency, and amount of drainage from the ostomy is recorded in the nurses' notes. In addition, the amount of drainage is recorded on the flow sheet and tallied in the total patient output for the shift.

29) Skin and Wounds

The skin assessment includes inspection for color and turgor, along with inspection for rashes, bruises, pressure ulcers, surgical wounds, and any other type of wound (such as bullet holes or knife wounds). Describe the size and location of the wound and whether the edges are approximated. Note if the wound is held together with sutures, staples, Steri-strips, or other material. A rash may indicate an allergy to a drug or other substance. Bruising may indicate problems with slowed blood clotting. Any type of wound or ulcer must be carefully assessed for infection, and notations must be made in the nurses' notes regarding the progress (or lack of progress) with healing.

When wounds are covered with a dressing, the nurse notes whether the dressing is clean, dry, and intact. Drainage is described for color and quantity. Sometimes a drain is placed inside the wound to facilitate removal of fluids and promote healing. The drainage tube is connected to a small fluid collection container such as a Jackson-Pratt bulb or a Hemovac. Jackson-Pratt and Hemovac are different brand names for drainage collection devices.

Skin assessments also involve checking for possible skin breakdown and development of pressure ulcers, also known pressure sores. The Braden scale or a similar rating form is used to predict the risk that a patient will develop a pressure ulcer; it is routinely completed for each patient. Factors predisposing a patient to pressure ulcers include:

- Inability to feel pain
- Skin that remains moist from perspiration or urine
- Lack of activity, such as when confined to bed
- Lack of mobility and ability to change body positions
- Poor nutrition
- The need to be moved up in bed, which can increase the risk of injury from friction and shear

JCAHO has specified that all patients be assessed for their *Risk of Impaired Skin Integrity*. Find the form used for assessing skin breakdown, and update it as needed based on the most current data you have collected on the patient.

30) Eyes, Ears, Nose, Throat

The nurse will record data about the patient's eyes, ears, nose, and throat, primarily related to the inspection for signs and symptoms of infection. Infections of these structures are common and bothersome. The signs and symptoms of infection include pain in the form of aching, soreness, or itching, along with redness, drainage, and edema.

Psychosocial and Cultural Assessment

The psychosocial and cultural assessment is very important. The focus of this chapter is on the assessment data that are gathered the night before clinical. Without talking with the patient, only a small amount of data may be collected regarding a patient's psychosocial/cultural background. The face sheet contains general information on religious preference, marital status, insurance information, and occupation. Psychosocial and cultural assessments are discussed

further in Chapter 6, which involves mapping of psychosocial problems.

31) Religious Preference

Religion is an important aspect of culture. Many patients practice a religion, such as Judaism, Buddhism, Islam, or Christianity. Of course, there are many variations within and between religious groups. Religious beliefs may influence a patient's view of sickness and the types of treatments that he finds acceptable and also commonly influence dietary practices and rituals associated with death and dying.

32) Marital Status

Marital status gives one indication of the structure of the patient's family and can be easily obtained the night before clinical. A major function of a healthy family is to be supportive. Spouses need to be included in the care plan, because they generally participate in the care of the patient in the health-care agency and in the home. Determining marital status is one element of the assessment of the social support system.

33) Health-Care Benefits and Insurance

The type of insurance the patient carries directly influences what will and will not be paid for regarding medications, treatments, surgeries, and other procedures. Insurance may or may not cover extended care or rehabilitation services. Knowing what will be covered by insurance is crucial to development of the care plan. A key question to think about is whether any community services are available to help the patient obtain services for which she cannot afford to herself.

34) Occupation

Occupation gives an indication of the patient's social status, income, and educational level. During your clinical day with the patient, you will need to assess when or if the patient will be able to return to work. By finding out the patient's occupation, you can begin thinking about how the person's ability to work will be affected by her health problems.

35) Emotional State

The emotional assessment is very important, so check the nurses' notes for notations about the patient's mood. Mood is a reflection of emotions, such as *Anxiety, Hopelessness, Powerlessness,* and *Ineffective Coping.* If you are able to meet your patient the day before clinical, you can make a direct observation of the patient's mood for your records. Does the patient appear happy? Sad? Quiet? Nervous? Record your impressions on the database.

Obtaining Standardized Forms

The night before clinical (or at the beginning of the next clinical day), gather all the standardized forms that pertain to your patient. These are printed materials that are used by the health-care agency on patients who have the same diagnosis as your patient.

Standardized Skin Assessment

The purpose of standardized skin assessment is to prevent pressure ulcers by estimating the patient's risk of developing them. The risk level is based on mental status, continence, mobility, activity, and nutrition. Those at highest risk have decreased levels of consciousness, incontinence, immobility, bedridden status, and inadequate intake of nutrients. You should know your patient's risk for developing an ulcer and plan to prevent this problem. Use the standardized form to estimate your patient's risk for pressure ulcer formation. You will include how to prevent pressure ulcers in the plan of care.

Standardized Falls–Risk Assessment

The purpose of the standardized falls–risk assessment is to prevent injury. Use the standardized falls–risk assessment form to estimate your patient's risk of falling. The risk to patients is based partly on mental status, with those patients who are confused and disoriented at highest risk. Another risk involves illness-related debilitation, which causes patients to be light-headed when standing, especially during the first 24 hours postoperatively. Patients with orthosta-

tic hypotension, visual impairments, mobility problems, and an unsteady gait are at risk as well. In addition, many patients take medications, such as sedatives and narcotics, which increase their risk for falling. Preventive measures related to falls should be incorporated into the nursing plan of care.

Standardized Nursing Care Plans

Many agencies have developed standardized nursing care plans for many common medical diagnoses. The care plans include the typical nursing diagnoses, expected patient outcomes, and nursing interventions.

Clinical Pathways

Clinical pathways (also known as critical pathways) are standard care plans that integrate all disciplines involved in a patient's care. This type of care planning has come about because of managed health care. The purpose of a clinical pathway is to coordinate services and decrease costs. Physicians, nurses, physical therapists, nutritionists, and other professionals jointly specify typical problems, interventions, and expected outcomes on a day-by-day basis for a specific disease or condition.

Pathways are in the process of development in many agencies, and you may or may not have pathways to follow. If pathways are being used, make sure you know exactly where your patient is on the pathway for the day you will be providing care. Analyze your patient's progress on the pathway to determine whether she is on time, behind the estimated schedule, or ahead of schedule. If she is ahead or behind, try to determine the reason for the variation.

Patient Education Materials

Patient education is an important aspect of nursing care. Many agencies have developed patient education materials; others use printed booklets. Audiovisual aids may also be available. Take these materials home with you, and study them. Integrate them into your plan of care. Be prepared to review educational materials with your patient as appropriate during the clinical day of care.

Communicating With Nursing Staff

Try to get as much patient information as possible on your own, and keep a list of questions about any information you cannot find on your patient. Then discuss that list in detail with your clinical faculty. Many students hesitate to bother nursing staff or other personnel in the agency when they are gathering data to prepare a plan of care. But most busy nurses do not mind answering a few thoughtful questions; after all, they were students, too, at one time. Keep in mind, however, that it is your responsibility to gather the relevant data. It is a learning experience for you to be searching out the information on your own, with clinical supervision from the faculty.

Once you have gathered information from the written records, find the nurse who is responsible for caring for your patient on the day of the assignment. Somewhere in the agency is an assignment sheet that shows all the patient assignments. When you find your patient's nurse, introduce yourself as a student nurse assigned to that patient on the following day. Then ask a very simple question, such as, "Is there anything special I should know about this patient?" Chances are you will get some good information that may not be written down anywhere. You may even be able to ask one or two more "quick" questions if the nurse has time. Many nurses are glad to have students' help in caring for their patients, and most do not mind answering brief questions if time allows. If the nurse is very busy, she may not have time to talk with you. If so, do not take it personally. The nurses do not know you, and they are busy. Save your remaining questions for your clinical faculty.

CHAPTER 2 SUMMARY

Gathering data is a time-consuming process, at least initially. It gets easier each time you do it, because you become more familiar with where to find the information. The only way you can develop a comprehensive plan of care is to make sure you have complete, accurate assessment data. Sound clinical judgments result from excellent assessments and data analysis.

Your patient profile database comes mainly from your review of patient records. Record keeping in health-care agencies is generally excellent, due to standards established by JCAHO and the ANA. In fact, data about patients are required to be accessible, recorded, and communicated.

The initial patient profile database is focused on pathophysiology and treatments, and it has psychological, social, and cultural components. This chapter describes the essential components of the basic patient profile database, the purpose of each component, and where the information is likely to be found in the medical records. The patient's current health problems and chronic health problems need to be identified, along with information derived from a head-to-toe physical assessment. In addition, treatments, medications, IV therapy, laboratory values, and diagnostic tests need to be identified and related to the patient's health problems. Diet and activity are also important aspects of treatment as well as the effects of health alterations on growth and development, emotional state, and the type of discomforts typically caused by the patient's health problem.

LEARNING ACTIVITIES

1. Go on a field trip with your clinical group and your clinical faculty to a hospital or outpatient setting. Locate and review the following records: patient charts and information contained in them, such as the face sheet, consent forms, laboratory data, and diagnostic test data; medication records; IV records; the Kardex; nursing flow sheets;

nursing assessments; and nurses' notes. Find out where to get the most recent information for each item. For example, perhaps the most recent laboratory data are in the front of the chart. This may vary from agency to agency and even from unit to unit within the agency.

2. After completing Exercise 1, work alone or with another student to complete a patient profile database, using Figure 2.1 with a real patient.

3. As you gather patient data, keep a list of abbreviations that were confusing and need clarification. Usually, each unit has its own set of abbreviations in addition to the standard abbreviations found in most textbooks. Hundreds of abbreviations are used inconsistently and thus create confusion. For example, DAT may mean diet as tolerated, and BKA may mean below-the-knee amputation. Write down anything that confuses you, and ask your faculty for clarification. Share your list with others in the clinical group.

4. Find out where the list of patient assignments is posted, and track down the staff nurse responsible for your patient. Be assertive, and ask how the patient is doing today. Go into the patient's room, and introduce yourself. Ask the patient how he is doing and if you can get him anything. Stay no longer than 5 minutes. If the patient asks for something you cannot do or provide, tell the nurse. The point of this exercise is to determine what you can assess about your patient's emotional state in just 5 brief minutes by listening to him and watching his nonverbal behavior.

REFERENCES

1. Nursing's Social Policy Statement, ed 2. American Nurses Association, nursesbooks.org, Washington, D.C., 2003.
2. Ericson, EH: Childhood and Society. Norton, New York, 1963 (reissued 1993).
3. Schuster, PM: Communication: The Key to the Therapeutic Relationship. FA Davis, Philadelphia, 2000.
4. Tannen, D: You Just Don't Understand: Women and Men in Conversation. Ballantine, New York, 1990.
5. Leeuwen, AM, Kranpitz, TR, and Smith, L: Laboratory and Diagnostic Tests with Nursing Implications, ed 2. FA Davis, Philadelphia, 2006.
6. Leeuwen, AM, Kranpitz, TR, and Smith L: op cit.

CONCEPT CARE MAPS: Grouping Clinical Data in a Meaningful Manner

OBJECTIVES

1. Identify the American Nurses Association (ANA) nursing standard of care related to organizing patient data.

2. Identify primary medical diagnoses.

3. Review patient profile data to determine general health problems.

4. Categorize patient profile data according to the patient's response to the health problem.

5. List primary assessments associated with the medical diagnosis.

6. Label nursing diagnoses.

7. Specify relationships between nursing diagnoses.

After gathering data, the next step in care planning is to develop the concept care map. The concept care map will contain the primary medical and nursing diagnoses for your patient and all the supporting data (disorders, medications, laboratory results, and treatments) categorized according to nursing diagnoses. In addition, relationships between diagnoses will be identified on the concept care map.

The basis of this chapter is the ANA standard of practice, which states that nursing diagnoses are to be derived from the health data.[1] Concept care maps promote critical analysis of health data in a way that increases the probability of formulating nursing diagnoses accurately. Students are sometimes too quick to put diagnostic labels on patients without data to support the diagnosis, resulting in diagnostic errors. Concept care maps help students organize data correctly and thus improve the accuracy of the nursing diagnoses.

You will follow three basic steps to develop a concept care map. These steps are based on meaningful learning theory and assimilation theory.[2,3] The first step is to diagram propositions. The second step is to arrange data in hierarchical order. The third step is to make meaningful associations between segments of the diagram. In this chapter, these theoretical steps will be defined with specific examples for application to nursing care plans.

Students are sometimes confused by the word "theory" or "theoretical." Theories are important because they explain phenomena. Meaningful learning theory and assimilation theory explain how you can increase your critical thinking abilities by mapping patient care concepts. A concept care map is a useful method for helping nursing students to reason clinically and formulate clinical judgments during analysis and organization of patient profile data. Students demonstrate critical thinking when organizing data logically in a concept care map. Critical thinking skills are used during the process of developing patient care maps.

This chapter is intended to give you practice in developing concept care maps for three different patient scenarios: a patient with diabetes, a surgical patient with a knee replacement, and a surgical patient with a mastectomy. Patient profile data are provided for each scenario. You will be guided step by step in completing a concept care map in the first scenario. Scenarios two and three are included in exercises at the end of the chapter for additional practice.

Scenario One: Database for Patient With Diabetes

Figure 3.1 contains data collected by a student nurse from a patient's records. The patient was hospitalized with newly diagnosed diabetes. The patient profile database is sketchy, but it contains all the information this student collected. Assume the student has not had much experience in collecting data, and this is her first patient assignment. Carefully review the information in Figure 3.1 to obtain some general ideas about the patient's problems that will be used for step 1 of concept care mapping. As you review the database, ignore the blank questions for now. The first step is to formulate initial impressions of the clinical patient profile data.

Step 1. Building a Framework

In step 1, you will diagram the framework of propositions. You must propose or state what you believe to be your patient's key problems based on the data you collected. The key problems are also known as the concepts. The framework is the diagram of the key problems. Do this step *before* you start to look up information in your reference materials. Start by centering the reason for admission to the health-care setting (often a medical diagnosis) on a sloppy copy (blank version) of your initial care map. The objective of doing a sloppy copy is to get the major problems down on a map where you can then critically think and analyze relationships between them. An example of a sloppy copy is shown in Figure 3.2.

Next, think about the big problems the medical diagnosis has created for this patient, based on the assessment data. He has problems with diet, nutrition, and elimination; he is anxious; he has not yet learned how to manage his care at home; and he has an ongoing medical problem of hypertension (blood pressure [BP]). Put these problems around the medical diagnosis, like spokes on a wagon wheel (Fig. 3.3)

The next task is to look up information on medical diagnoses, medications, and treatments. The reason is to develop a general understanding of what is wrong with the patient and what is being done by the physician to correct the patient's problems. Assume you are in your first clinical course with your first patient assignment and that you are learning assessment and fundamentals of nursing, including medication administration.

It is now appropriate to attempt to answer some questions about the information in Figure 3.1. You will need to use course textbooks and software to look up information. Reference materials may include a medical dictionary, a man-

Student Name: **PMT**

1) Date of Care: **3/23**	2) Patient Initials: **ET**	3) Age: **80** (face sheet)	3) Growth and Development **Ego integrity vs. Despair**	4) Gender: **M** (face sheet)	5) Admission Date: (face sheet) **3/21**

6) Reason for hospitalization (face sheet): Describe reason for hospitalization: (expand on back of page) *Medical Dx:* **Diabetes Type II** *Pathophysiology:* All signs and symptoms: *Highlight those your patient exhibits* **Polydipsia, polyphagia, polyuria, weakness, increased blood glucose, increased glycohemoglobin, glycosuria**	7) Chronic illnesses (physician's history and physical notes in chart; nursing intake assessment and Kardex) **Hypertension**
8) Surgical procedures (consent forms and Kardex): Describe surgical procedure (expand on back of page) Name of surgical procedure: **NA** *Describe surgery:*	

9) ADVANCE DIRECTIVES (NURSE'S ADMISSION ASSESSMENTS):

Living will: ☐ Yes ☐ No	Power of attorney: ☐ Yes ☐ No	Do not resuscitate (DNR) order (Kardex): ☐ Yes ☐ No

10) LABORATORY DATA:

Test	Normal Values	Admission 3/21	Date/Time 3/23	Date/Time	Reason for Abnormal Values
White blood cells (WBCs)					
Red blood cells (RBCs)					
Hemoglobin (Hgb)					
Hematocrit (Hct)					
Platelets					
Prothrombin time (PT)					
International normalized ratio (INR)					
Activated partial thromboplastin time (Aptt)					
Sodium Na					
Potassium K					
Chloride Cl					
Glucose (FBS/BS)		450	120		
Hemoglobin A1C		12%			
Cholesterol		240			
Blood Urea Nitrogen (BUN)					
Creatinine					
Urine analysis (UA)		3+sugar			
Pre-albumin					
Albumin					
Calcium Ca					
Phosphate					
Bilirubin					
Alkaline phosphatase					
SGOT-Serum glutamic-oxyloacetic transaminase					
AST-Serum glutamic pyruvic transaminase					
CK					
CK MB					
Troponin					
B-natriuretic peptide BNP					
pH					
pCO_2					
pO_2					
HCO_3					

11) DIAGNOSTIC TESTS

Chest x-ray:	EKG:	Other abnormal reports:
Sputum or Blood Culture:	Other:	Other:

12) MEDICATIONS

List medications and times of administration (medication administration record and check the drawer in the carts for spelling). Include over-the-counter (OTC) products/herbal medicines.

		qam 0730	qam 0900	q4h pm	
Times Due		qam 0730	qam 0900	q4h pm	
Brand Name		**Humulin N**	**Diovan**	**tylenol**	
Generic Name		**NPH Insulin**	**Valsartan**	**Acetaminophen**	
Dose		**35U**	**80mg**	**650mg**	
Administration Route					
Classification					
Action					
Reason This Patient is Receiving					
Pharmacokinetics		O P D 1/2 M E	O P D 1/2 M E	O P D 1/2 M E	O P D 1/2 M E
Contraindications					
Major Adverse Side Effects					
Nursing Implications					
Pt/Family Teaching					

Developed by P. Testa, YSU

ALLERGIES/PAINS

13) Allergies: Type of Reaction: (medication administration record):	14) When was the last time pain medication given? (medication administration record)
14) Where is the pain? (nurse's notes)	14) How much pain is the patient in on a scale 0-10? (nurse's notes, flow sheet):

TREATMENTS

15) List treatments (Kardex): Rationale for treatments:
Glucometer qid ac & hs
VS q4h
Position changes q2h
Ted hose
IS q1h while awake
C&DB q1h while awake

16) Support services (Kardex) What do support services provide for the patient? **Dietitian and Diabetes Educator**

17) What does the consultant do for the patient?:

18) DIET/FLUIDS

Type of Diet (Kardex): **1800 ADA**	Restrictions (Kardex): **No sugar added**	Gag reflex intact: [X] Yes ☐ No	Appetite: [X] Good ☐ Fair ☐ Poor	Breakfast **100** %	Lunch **100** %	Dinner **100** %

What type of diet is this?:

What types of foods are included in this diet and what foods should be avoided?:

Circle Those Problems That Apply:

Prior 24 hours Fluid intake: (Oral & IV) **2200** Fluid output **1800** (flow sheet)	• Problems: swallowing, chewing, dentures (nurse's notes) • Needs assistance with feeding (nurse's notes) • Nausea or vomiting (nurse's notes) • Overhydrated or dehydrated (evaluate total intake and output on flow sheet
Tube feedings: Type and rate (Kardex)	• Belching: • Other: _____

19) INTRAVENOUS FLUIDS (IV therapy record)

Type and Rate: **NA**	IV dressing dry, no edema, redness of site: ☐ Yes ☐ No	Other:

52

20) ELIMINATION (flow sheet)

Last bowel movement:	Foley/condom catheter: ☐ Yes ☐ No

Circle Those Problems That Apply:

- Bowel: constipation diarrhea flatus incontinence belching
- Urinary: hesitancy frequency burning incontinence odor
- Other: _____
- What is causing the problem in elimination? __**History of polyuria**_____

21) ACTIVITY (Kardex, flow sheet)

Ability to walk (gait): **Unsteady**	Type of activity orders: **OOB/chair**	Use of assistance devices: cane, walker, crutches, prosthesis:	Falls-risk assessment rating:
No. of side rails required (flow sheet) **2**	Restraints (flow sheet): ☐ Yes ☒ No	Weakness ☒ Yes ☐ No	Trouble sleeping (nurse's notes): ☐ Yes ☐ No

What does activity order mean?: _____

Why isn't the patient up ad lib?: _____

Would the problem cause weakness?: _____

PHYSICAL ASSESSMENT DATA

22) BP (flow sheet): **132/92**	2) TPR (flow sheet): **98.4-77-18**	23) Height: __**5' 10"**__ Weight: __**174**__ (nursing intake assessments)

24) NEUROLOGICAL/MENTAL STATUS:

LOC: alert and oriented to person, place, time (A&O x 3), confused, etc. **A&Ox3**	Speech: clear, appropriate/inappropriate **Clear**
Pupils: PERRLA **PERRLA**	Sensory deficits for vision/hearing/taste/ smell **Glasses**

25) MUSCULOSKELETAL STATUS:

Bones, joints, muscles (fractures, contractures, arthritis, spinal curvatures, etc):	Extremity (temperature, edema (pitting vs. nonpitting) & sensation)
Motor: ROM x 4 extremities **Full ROM**	
Ted hose/plexi pulses/compression devices: type:	Casts, splint, collar, brace:

26) CARDIOVASCULAR SYSTEM:

Pulses (radial, pedal) (to touch or with Doppler): **3+ pedals & radials**	Capillary refill (<3s): ☐ Yes ☐ No	
Neck vein (distention):	Sounds: S1, S2, regular, irregular: Apical rate: **76 rrr**	Any chest pain:

27) RESPIRATORY SYSTEM:

Depth, rate, rhythm: **20**	Use of accessory muscles:	Cyanosis:	Sputum color, amount:	Cough: productive nonproductive	Breath sounds: clear, rales, wheezes **Clear**
Use of oxygen: nasal cannula, mask, trach collar:	Flow rate of oxygen:	Oxygen humidification: ☐ Yes ☐ No		Pulse oximeter: _____ % oxygen saturation	Smoking: ☐ Yes ☐ No

28) GASTROINTESTINAL SYSTEM

Abdominal pain, tenderness, guarding; distention, soft, firm: **Soft, nondistended**	Bowel sounds x 4 quadrants: **Present 4 quads**	NG tube: describe drainage
Ostomy: describe stoma site and stools:	Other:	

29) SKIN AND WOUNDS:

Color, turgor: **Pink**	Rash, bruises:	Describe wounds (size, locations):	Edges approximated: ☐ Yes ☐ No	Type of wound drains:
Characteristics of drainage:	Dressings (clean, dry, intact):	Sutures, staples, steri-strips, other:	Risk for pressure ulcer assessment rating:	Other:

30) EYES, EARS, NOSE, THROAT (EENT):

Eyes: redness, drainage, edema, ptosis	Ears: drainage	Nose: redness, drainage, edema	Throat: sore
Psychosocial and Cultural Assessment			

31) Religious preference (face sheet) **Catholic**	32) Marital status (face sheet) **Widower**	33) Health care benefits and insurance (face sheet): **Blue Cross/Blue Shield**
34) Occupation (face sheet) **Retired**	35) Emotional state (nurse's notes) **Anxious about giving insulin and following diet**	

● Figure 3.1   Patient profile database. Scenario 1: Patient newly diagnosed with diabetes.

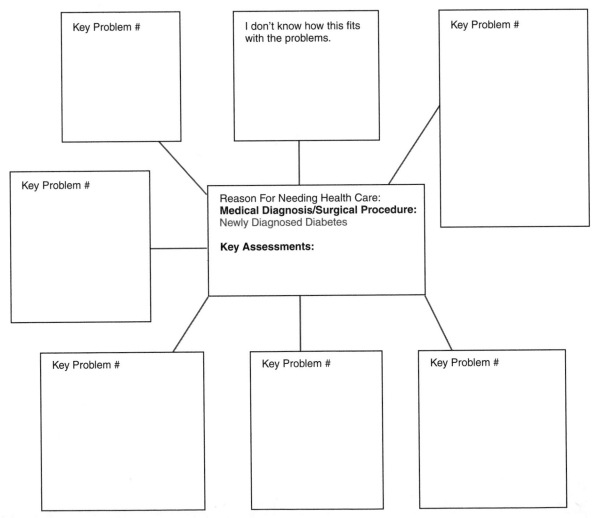

● Figure 3.2   Sloppy copy (preconference). Carry in your pocket at all times!

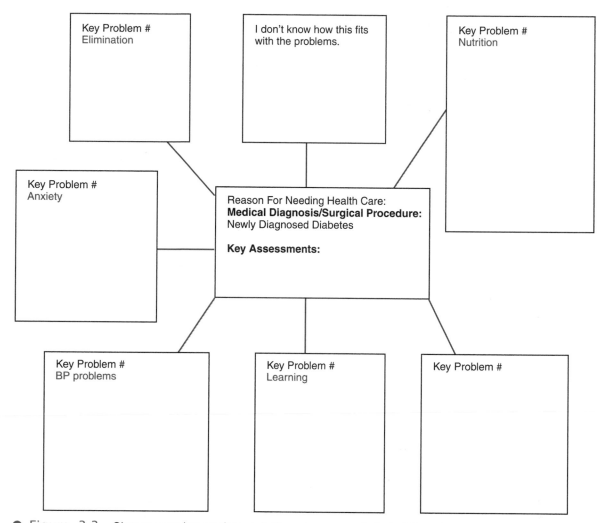

● Figure 3.3   Sloppy copy (preconference). Carry in your pocket at all times!

ual of laboratory and diagnostic procedures, a book on nutrition therapy, a drug handbook or pharmacology book, a standardized care plan book, a fundamentals textbook, and a medical-surgical text book. You may use PDA software programs and Internet sites, which decrease the amount of time required to research materials, such as computerized drug guides[4] or computerized nursing care plans.[5] There is also an Internet site, *www.ask.com*, to learn about any topic. Go to the site, ask any question, and you will get an answer. For example, go to the site, ask for patient education for diabetes, and you will find all kinds of information in an instant. Be careful that the information you retain is from a reliable source and the information is based on research.

Looking Up Information

For this patient, you will need to look up information about drugs, laboratory and diagnostic tests, diet, and medical diagnoses.

Drugs

Start by looking up drugs. There are only three for this patient: Humulin N (NPH insulin), Diovan (valsartan), and Tylenol (acetaminophen). You may be thinking, "Why start with drugs?" Medication administration is one of the most dangerous things nurses do, and it is a primary focus of fundamentals courses. Therefore, before you use your energy looking up everything else, invest some time when your mind is fresh, reading and taking some notes on the drugs. Patient education with regard to drugs is a key nursing responsibility. Determine the type of information the patient needs to know about taking his drugs properly at home.

Laboratory and Diagnostic Tests

Next, read about the laboratory and diagnostic tests in a laboratory and diagnostic procedures manual. Medication administration is often based on laboratory values. There is a direct relationship between the laboratory values and the patient's medication. You must identify those relationships. Make sure you know the most up-to-date laboratory values before you administer drugs. Also, patient teaching is needed regarding laboratory tests, so you must identify what the patient needs to know about the diagnostic tests that have been ordered.

Diet

Obtain information on the patient's prescribed diet. How is the diet related to the medical diagnosis? What patient education is needed regarding diet? What is a sample menu for the patient? If you have a nutritional therapy book, at least one chapter will be devoted to diabetes. If you do not have a nutrition book, use the *www.ask.com* Web site. Ask for information about diabetic diets.

Medical Diagnoses/Chronic Illnesses

Find information about the patient's medical diagnoses. Your fundamentals text may not offer much help because many such books contain little disease-specific information. The aim of a fundamentals text is to teach foundational skills essential for providing care of basic human needs. Fundamentals courses typically do not cover specific aspects of medical-surgical nursing care. Therefore, you may find a medical dictionary helpful for defining the disease and providing symptoms, etiology, complications, treatments, prognosis, and nursing implications.

The most detailed information about diseases can be found in a medical-surgical nursing text. In fact, it is a good investment to buy a medical-surgical text ahead of time so you can use the book as a reference in your fundamentals course. You may find certain Web sites helpful as well, such as those listed in Box 3.1.

Other helpful references include standardized care plan guidelines and clinical pathways. These may be obtained from the health-care agency or from standardized care planning manuals.[6] Standardized care plans include patient goals, patient outcomes, nursing interventions, and rationales. Clinical pathways also integrate the services of other health professionals in attaining patient goals. These are general guidelines, not specific to a particular patient. The concept care map that you develop will be specific to your patient on the day you provide care for him.

As you review standardized plans and pathways, you must sort through all the possible nursing diagnoses, goals, objectives, and interventions; then you must determine what is appropriate for the day you are assigned to care for the patient. This is called individualizing the plan of care. This is difficult at first, but with practice and experience you will get better at it. An important point to remember as you review informa-

Box 3.1	WEB SITES: GATHERING INFORMATION
American Heart Association	*www.americanheart.org*
Arthritis Foundation	*www.arthritis.org*
National Cancer Institute	*www.cancernet.nic.nih.gov*
American Diabetes Association	*www.diabetes.org*
Immunization Action Coalition	*www.immunize.org*
American Lung Association	*www.lungusa.org*
Mental Health InfoSource	*www.mhsource.org*
Nephron Information Center	*www.nephron.com*
Neurosciences on the Internet	*www.neuroguide.com*
National Organization for Rare Disorders	*www.rarediseases.org*

tion from standardized plans is that you must determine what is most relevant to the patient at the time you are assigned to care for him.

Preventing Falls and Skin Breakdown

The next part of step 1 in building a concept map for your diabetic patient is to analyze his risk for falls and skin breakdown. Preventing falls and skin breakdown is fundamental to competent nursing care. The Joint Commission on Accreditation of Healthcare Organizations (JCAHO) requires that all patients be evaluated for falls and skin breakdown; thus, each agency will have assessment forms for this task. Samples of assessment forms with data from the case study in this chapter are shown in Figures 3.4 and 3.5. These have been filled out based on patient profile data and on what is known about patients with diabetes. Thus, the specifics of the data collected and the general information for a patient with diabetes are used to complete the assessments. You must rate your patient for falls and skin breakdown based on the most current information you obtained on the patient.

When assessing the patient's risk of falling, as shown in Figure 3.4, consider that the patient is older than 60 years, he is weak, he has had problems with urinary frequency, and he is taking an antihypertensive.[7] By looking up information, you may conclude that his weakness is from inadequate nutrition and dehydration. Urinary frequency is associated with polyuria; the antihypertensive drug may contribute to orthostatic hypotension; and decreased muscle tone and strength may be associated with aging. Therefore, this patient is at risk for a fall. Write the total fall risk score in the upper right box of the assessment form, and then write in the upper right box of the assessment form your clinical judgment that the patient is at risk for falling.

Next, assess the patient's risk for development of pressure sores. Each patient is assessed for potential problems in developing skin breakdown. This breakdown is termed a pressure sore, or pressure ulcer. Figure 3.5 shows the Braden Scale for Predicting Pressure Sore Risk.[8] To assess risk, score the patient on each of the six subscales, and total the points. The maximum score is 23, which indicates little or no risk. A score between 10 and 16 indicates a risk of pres-

sure ulcer. A score of 9 or less indicates a high risk of pressure ulcer.

How would you rate the diabetic patient in this scenario? Based on data from the patient's profile, the patient does not have any sensory impairments (4 points); is probably rarely moist (4 points); probably walks occasionally (3 points); probably has slightly limited mobility from being only out of bed and in a chair (OOB/chair) (3 points); has excellent nutrition (4 points); and has a potential problem with friction and shear (2 points). He has 20 of 23 points based on the evidence provided in the patient profile database. Thus, he has a low risk for developing a pressure ulcer. Write the total pressure sore risk score in the box in the lower right corner of the assessment form, and then write your clinical judgment that the patient is at low risk of developing a pressure sore in this box.

There are many assessments that you may need to do, depending on the course you are taking and the condition of the patient. For example, there is an assessment for pain shown in Figure 3.6 and an assessment for neurological functioning shown in Figure 3.7.

At this point, you have completed the patent profile database and researched basic information about the disease and its treatment. It is now time to categorize the data you have gathered under the basic problems you identified on your map. All the pieces of data must be organized into a hierarchical and comprehensive pattern.

Step 2: Mapping the Hierarchy

According to educational theory, concept maps are hierarchical graphical organizers. A hierarchy is a tiered series of consecutive classes or groups. For example, one hierarchy in biology is the classification of living things into kingdom, phylum, class, order, family, genus, and species. Subconcepts are organized in a pattern under major concepts, to facilitate understanding of relationships and to organize information. The graph of the hierarchy is a picture or map of the organized relationships between concepts and subconcepts.

In concept care mapping, the subconcepts are the specific pieces of data that were collected about the patient and that support the major problems you identified on the spokes of the wheel surrounding the reason for admission to

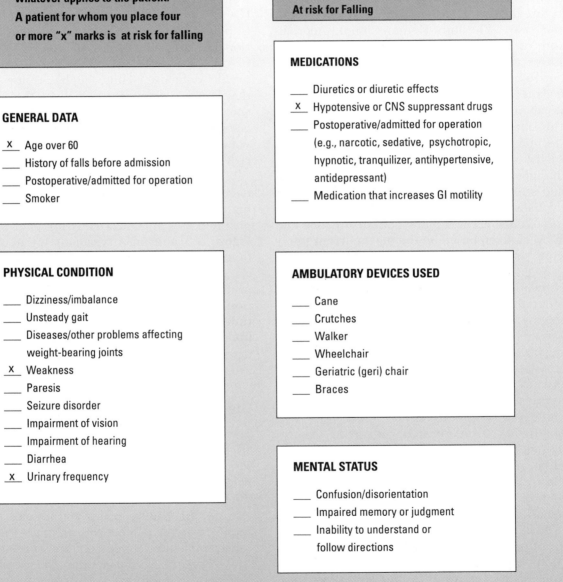

RISK FOR FALLS ASSESSMENT

DIRECTIONS: Place an "x" in front of elements that apply to your patient. Based on the assessment, check whatever applies to the patient. A patient for whom you place four or more "x" marks is at risk for falling

Total Score __4__   Clinical Judgment

At risk for Falling

MEDICATIONS

___ Diuretics or diuretic effects
_X_ Hypotensive or CNS suppressant drugs
___ Postoperative/admitted for operation
    (e.g., narcotic, sedative, psychotropic,
    hypnotic, tranquilizer, antihypertensive,
    antidepressant)
___ Medication that increases GI motility

GENERAL DATA

_X_ Age over 60
___ History of falls before admission
___ Postoperative/admitted for operation
___ Smoker

PHYSICAL CONDITION

___ Dizziness/imbalance
___ Unsteady gait
___ Diseases/other problems affecting
    weight-bearing joints
_X_ Weakness
___ Paresis
___ Seizure disorder
___ Impairment of vision
___ Impairment of hearing
___ Diarrhea
_X_ Urinary frequency

AMBULATORY DEVICES USED

___ Cane
___ Crutches
___ Walker
___ Wheelchair
___ Geriatric (geri) chair
___ Braces

MENTAL STATUS

___ Confusion/disorientation
___ Impaired memory or judgment
___ Inability to understand or
    follow directions

● Figure 3.4   Assessing risk for falls. Assess prior to clinical day. (From Brians, LK, et al: The development of the RISK tool for fall prevention. Rehabilitation Nursing 1991:16[2]:67, with permission.)

Directions: Add up the total points, a perfect score is 23. A high score means lower risk for pressure ulcer. A low score means higher risk for pressure ulcer.

BRADEN SCALE >>> *FOR PREDICTING PRESSURE SORE RISK*

Patient's Name:	Evaluator's Name:	Date of Assessment:

	1	**2**	**3**	**4**
SENSORY PERCEPTION Ability to respond meaningfully to pressure-related discomfort	**Completely limited:** Unresponsive (does not moan, flinch, or grasp) to painful stimuli, due to diminished level of consciousness or sedation, OR limited ability to feel pain over most of the body surface.	**Very Limited:** Responds only to painful stimuli. Cannot communicate discomfort except by moaning or restlessness, OR has a sensory impairment which limits the ability to feel pain or discomfort over 1/2 of the body.	**Slightly Limited:** Responds to verbal commands but cannot always communicate discomfort or need to be turned, OR has a sensory impairment which limits ability to feel pain or discomfort in 1 or 2 extremities.	**No Impairment:** Responds to verbal commands. Has no sensory deficit which would limit ability to feel or voice pain or discomfort.
MOISTURE Degree to which skin is exposed to moisture	**Constantly Moist:** Skin is kept moist almost constantly by perspiration, urine, etc. Dampness is detected every time patient is moved or turned.	**Moist:** Skin is often but not always moist. Linen must be changed at least once a shift.	**Occasionally Moist:** Skin is occasionally moist, requiring an extra linen change approximately once a day.	**Rarely Moist:** Skin is usually dry; linen requires changing only at routine intervals.
ACTIVITY Degree of physical activity	**Bedfast:** Confined to bed.	**Chairfast:** Ability to walk severely limited or nonexistent. Cannot bear own weight and/or must be assisted into chair or wheelchair.	**Walks Occasionally:** Walks occasionally during day but for very short distances, with or without assistance. Spends majority of each shift in bed or chair.	**Walks Frequently:** Walks outside the room at least twice a day and inside room at least once every 2 hours during walking hours.
MOBILITY Ability to change and control body position	**Completely Immobile:** Does not make even slight changes in body or extremity position without assistance.	**Very Limited:** Makes occasional slight changes in body or extremity position but unable to make frequent or significant changes independently.	**Slightly Limited:** Makes frequent though slight changes in body or extremity position independently.	**No Limitations:** Makes major and frequent changes in position without assistance.
NUTRITION Usual food intake pattern	**Very Poor:** Never eats a complete meal. Rarely eats more than 1/3 of any food offered. Eats 2 servings or less of protein (meat or dairy products) per day. Takes fluids poorly. Does not take a liquid dietary supplement, OR is NPO and/or maintained on clear liquids or IVs for more than 5 days.	**Probably Inadequate:** Rarely eats a complete meal and generally eats only about 1/2 of any food offered. Protein intake includes 3 servings of meat or dairy products per day. Occasionally will take a dietary supplement, OR receives less than optimum amount of liquid diet or tube feeding.	**Adequate:** Eats over half of meals. Eats a total of 4 servings of protein (meat, dairy products) each day. Occasionally will refuse a meal, but will usually take a supplement if offered, OR is on a tube feeding or TPN regimen, which probably meets most of nutritional needs.	**Excellent:** Eats most of every meal. Never refuses a meal. Usually eats a total of 4 or more servings of meat and dairy products. Occasionally eats between meals. Does not require supplementation.
FRICTION AND SHEAR	**Problem:** Requires moderate to maximum assistance in moving. Complete lifting without sliding against sheets is impossible. Frequently slides down in bed or chair, requiring frequent repositioning with maximum assistance. Spasticity, contractures, or agitation leads to almost constant friction.	**Potential Problem:** Moves feebly or requires minimum assistance. During a move skin probably slides to some extent against the sheets, chair, restraints, or other devices. Maintains relatively good position in chair or bed most of the time but occasionally slides down.	**No Apparent Problem:** Moves in bed and in chair independently and has sufficient muscle strength to lift up completely during move. Maintains good position in bed or chair at all times.	**Total Points:** _____ **Clinical Judgment** _____ _____ _____ _____

● Figure 3.5   Braden Scale for Predicting Pressure Ulcer Assessment. (From Braden, B, and Bergstrom, N: In Bryant, RA [ed]: Acute and Chronic Wounds: Nursing Management. Mosby, St. Louis, 1992.)

Initial Pain Assessment Tool

Date _____

Patient's Name _____ Age _____ Room _____

Diagnosis _____ Physician _____

Nurse _____

1. LOCATION: Patient or nurse mark drawing.

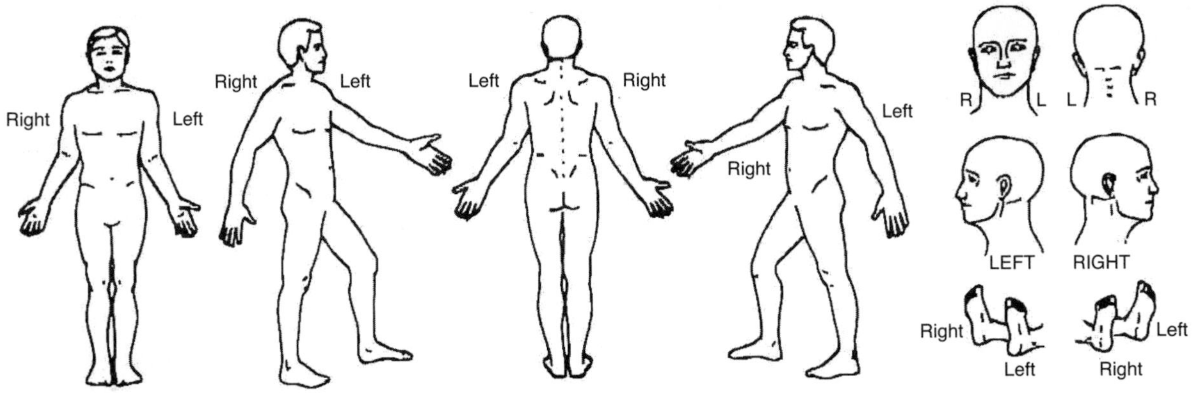

2. INTENSITY: Patient rates the pain. Scale used _____
   Present: _____
   Worst pain gets: _____
   Best pain gets: _____
   Acceptable level of pain: _____

3. QUALITY: (Use patient's own words, e.g., prick, ache, burn, throb, pull, sharp) _____

   _____

4. ONSET, DURATION, VARIATIONS, RHYTHMS: _____
   _____

5. MANNER OF EXPRESSING PAIN: _____
   _____
   _____

6. WHAT RELIEVES THE PAIN? _____
   _____
   _____

7. WHAT CAUSES OR INCREASES THE PAIN? _____
   _____
   _____

8. EFFECTS OF PAIN: (Note decreased function, decreased quality of life.)
   Accompanying symptoms (e.g., nausea) _____
   Sleep _____
   Appetite _____
   Physical activity _____
   Relationship with others (e.g., irritability) _____
   Emotions (e.g., anger, suicidal, crying) _____
   Concentration _____
   Other _____

9. OTHER COMMENTS: _____

10. PLAN: _____
    _____
    _____

● Figure 3.6 Initial pain assessment tool assessment during clinical day. (DeLaune, S, and Ladner, P. Fundamentals of Nursing: Standards and Practice. Delmar Thomson Learning, Albany, NY, 2002.)

Clinical Judgment _____

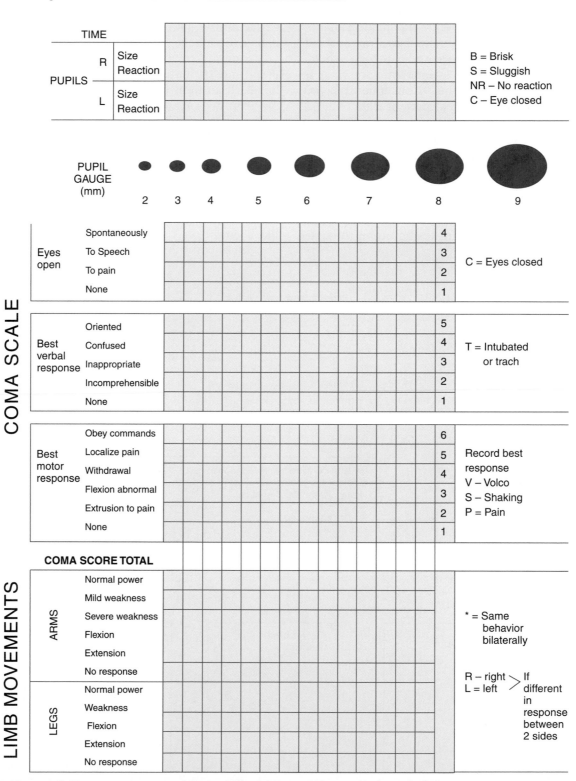

● Figure 3.7   Assessing neurological status (Glasgow Coma Scale).

the health-care setting. The subconcepts are the clinical pathological signs and symptoms the patient displayed, treatments, medications, laboratory data, and chronic illness data. You must sift through the data once more and categorize them.

Keep in mind that a concept care map is based on actual problems. Consequently, you should categorize only real patient data. This is one reason why it is important for you to look up information on the patient's disease, drugs, treatments, surgery, and so on before categorizing the data; that way, you have general knowledge of the main treatments for the primary medical diagnosis and surgical procedures. The problems that extend out from the central reason for admission will become nursing diagnoses based on the defi-

nitions and classifications of the North American Nursing Diagnosis Association (NANDA).[9] Categorize all the data you have *before* assigning any diagnostic labels.

Start by reviewing the physical assessment data, and try categorizing them in appropriate boxes. If an item belongs in more than one box, put it in two or more places. If you do not know where an item goes, place it in the central box labeled "I don't know how this fits with the problems."). This is a very important box. There are times when you may find medications the patient should not be taking or treatments the patient should not be receiving and need to be discontinued. At this stage your map should look like Figure 3.8.

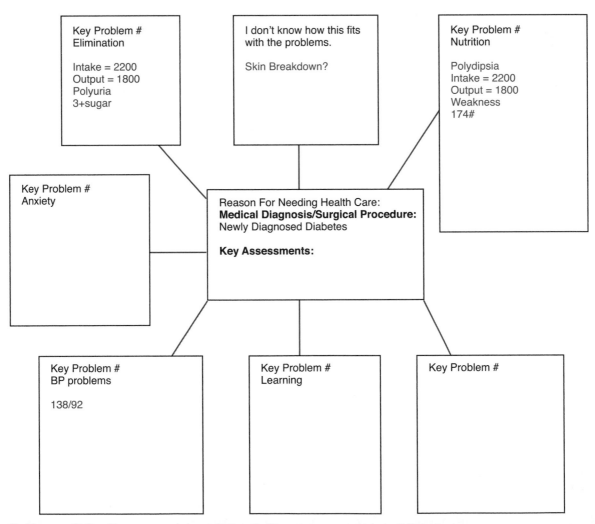

● Figure 3.8   Sloppy copy (preconference). Carry in your pocket at all times!

Now try to add remaining pieces of data items into your boxes. For example, add information about drugs (Humulin N, Diovan, Tylenol), laboratory test results (serum glucose 450 down to 120, glycosylated hemoglobin = 12%, cholesterol = 240, urine 3+ sugar), treatments (glucometer-Accucheck, VS qid), diet (1800 American Diabetes Association [ADA], no added sugar), activity (OOB/chair, risk of falls), and psycho-social-cultural data (anxiety about injections and diet, widower). Now your map might look like Figure 3.9.

You must be able to explain why you put each item in the box you selected based on what your reading about the pathophysiology, your monitoring, and treatment of the disease.

A number of items are listed at the top of the map in the box titled "I don't know how this fits with the problems," items that do not seem to fit any of the other boxes. If you look at these items as a group, they suggest that the patient is not as mobile as he should be, and he has a risk of falling. This realization warrants adding another box to your map to address the patient's mobility problem. The symptom of weakness also goes along with this problem of mobility. Therefore, a key problem is immobility; this problem is placed in a separate box. See Figure 3.10 for an example.

Suppose you are still not sure about the remaining items in the "I don't know how this fits with the problems" box: acetaminophen, widower, and skin breakdown. This means you

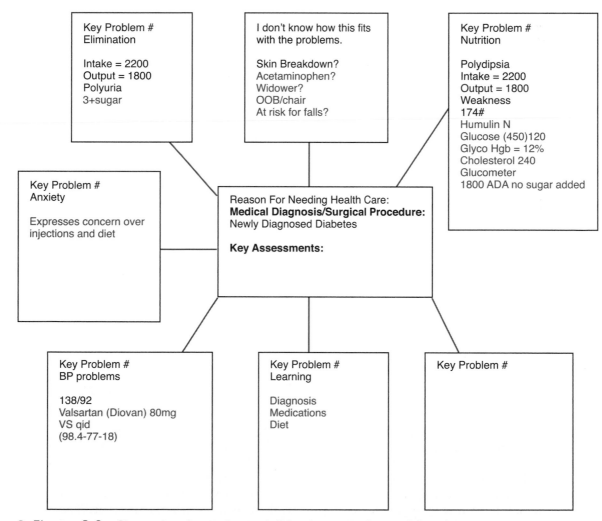

● Figure 3.9   Sloppy copy (preconference). Carry in your pocket at all times!

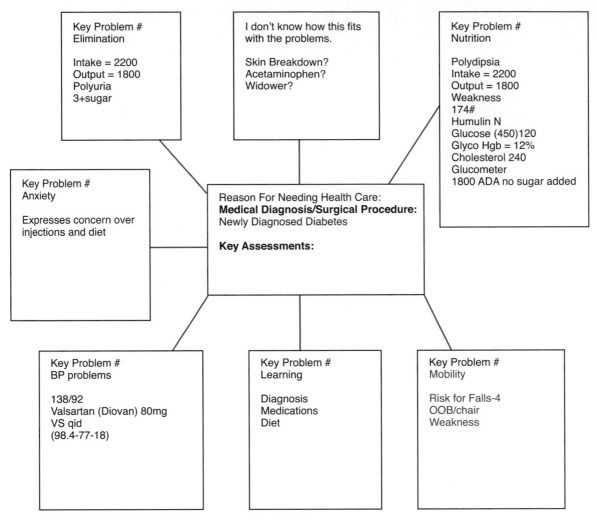

Key Problem #
Elimination

Intake = 2200
Output = 1800
Polyuria
3+sugar

I don't know how this fits
with the problems.

Skin Breakdown?
Acetaminophen?
Widower?

Key Problem #
Nutrition

Polydipsia
Intake = 2200
Output = 1800
Weakness
174#
Humulin N
Glucose (450)120
Glyco Hgb = 12%
Cholesterol 240
Glucometer
1800 ADA no sugar added

Key Problem #
Anxiety

Expresses concern over
injections and diet

Reason For Needing Health Care:
Medical Diagnosis/Surgical Procedure:
Newly Diagnosed Diabetes

Key Assessments:

Key Problem #
BP problems

138/92
Valsartan (Diovan) 80mg
VS qid
(98.4-77-18)

Key Problem #
Learning

Diagnosis
Medications
Diet

Key Problem #
Mobility

Risk for Falls-4
OOB/chair
Weakness

● Figure 3.10   Sloppy copy (preconference). Carry in your pocket at all times!

have not collected enough data to make decisions about those items, and you need to do more assessment when you meet with the patient the next day. For example, you need to find out whether the acetaminophen was prophylactic and never used. Did the patient have pain somewhere? Was he running a temperature? What type of social support does he have as a widower? The answer to this question could have major implications if the patient has no one at home to help him accomplish the self-care tasks the patient cannot accomplish on his own. He may need nursing home placement or home health care. What about the skin breakdown? The patient does not have any specific problems noted in the data, but from your reading you may have noted that diabetics have trouble with cir-

culation and sensation in their legs and feet, making them prone to skin breakdown. In addition, their wounds heal slowly. The patient needs to be taught foot care and methods to prevent skin breakdown.

Adding Assessments for Primary Medical Diagnoses

Now that you have most of your patient data arranged on your concept care map, you should add key assessments to the central box that contains the reason (the medical diagnosis) for admission to the health-care setting. These are important assessments that you will focus on while you are with the patient. The results of these assessments will tell you whether the patient is making progress toward a healthier state in which his diabetes is under control.

In a patient with diabetes, the key assessments consist of watching for hypoglycemia or hyperglycemia and assessing blood glucose levels. Hypoglycemia typically causes weakness, dizziness, sluggishness, hunger, irritability, sweating, paleness, a rapid heart rate, tremors, headache, and changes in mental functioning, such as confusion. The potential for hypoglycemia in the hospital setting is high until food intake, exercise, and the amount of insulin the patient receives are in careful balance. The classic signs of hyperglycemia and ketosis are polydipsia (excessive thirst), polyuria (excessive urination), and polyphagia (excessive appetite).

The most important problem to watch for in this patient is an insulin reaction. When giving the patient his insulin, make sure you know his blood glucose level and that he is going to eat if you are giving a pre-meal dose. Always monitor vital signs. The center of the care map should look like Figure 3.11.

Labeling Nursing Diagnoses

Remember to attach nursing diagnoses labels to problems *after* carefully considering all the data. Many students have a tendency to select nursing diagnoses too quickly, without first looking at and organizing the data. The net result of making quick decisions about diagnoses is that

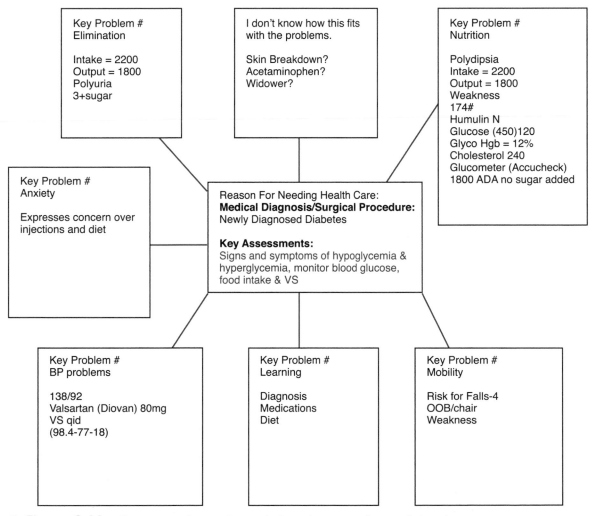

● Figure 3.11   Sloppy copy (preconference). Carry in your pocket at all times!

the diagnoses are often wrong. Therefore, take time to look at the data before you leap into the diagnoses.

Assigning correct diagnoses is essential to developing an individualized plan of care that includes appropriate goals, outcome objectives, and interventions specific to the day you are assigned to care for the patient. It will be impossible to develop an individualized plan if you have not accurately identified and prioritized the patient's specific problems. Once you have done so, it is relatively easy to find information on what to do to correct those problems. Developing the plan of care once the correct diagnoses are made is the subject of Chapter 4.

Nursing diagnoses are statements that describe a patient's actual or potential responses to health problems or life processes that the nurse is licensed and competent to treat.[10-15] Nursing diagnoses are focused on the patient's responses to a health problem. In contrast, medical diagnoses are focused on the health problem itself, based on the signs and symptoms related to the pathophysiology of the disease. Medical and nursing diagnoses are inextricably linked, and you—as the nurse—must recognize the linkages. The linkages between the medical and nursing diagnoses are clearly shown by the lines between the medical and nursing diagnoses on the concept map. The nursing diagnoses flow outward from the primary medical diagnosis like spokes on a wheel. You will continue to grow in your knowledge of nursing diagnoses and medical diagnoses with each day of clinical experience.

For the medical diagnosis of diabetes, the resulting general problems that you identified are elimination, nutrition, learning, anxiety, blood pressure problems, and immobility. These are the problems that you believe to be the patient's responses to the health problem of diabetes. In concept care mapping, the focus is on actual problems, real data, not potential problems.

In the NANDA system, the nursing diagnoses have been placed into a framework that groups them in categories and makes them easy to locate. Nursing diagnoses have been arranged according to Maslow's hierarchy of self-actualization needs (see Appendix A), which include:

- Self-esteem
- Love and belonging

- Safety and security
- Physiological needs[16]

They have also been organized according to Gordon's Functional Health Patterns (see Appendix B), which include:

- Health-perception–health-management pattern
- Nutritional-metabolic pattern
- Elimination pattern
- Activity-exercise pattern
- Sleep-rest pattern
- Cognitive-perceptual pattern
- Self-perception–self-concept pattern
- Role-relationship pattern
- Sexuality-reproductive pattern
- Coping-stress tolerance pattern
- Value-belief pattern[17]

A third popular framework is NANDA's Human Response Patterns, which include:

- Exchanging
- Communicating
- Relating
- Valuing
- Choosing
- Moving
- Perceiving
- Knowing and feeling[18]

Each nursing diagnosis you select for your map must be based on an accurate assessment of the patient's problems. Use the appendices of this book to locate possible diagnoses for the problems you identified. Review Maslow's Hierarchy (Appendix A), Gordon's Functional Health Patterns (Appendix B), Doenges' and Moorhouse's Diagnostic Division (Appendix C), and NANDA's classification system (Appendix D).

Each of the problem areas identified for the diabetic patient scenario will be described below, with an explanation of the critical thinking that was needed to determine the final nursing diagnosis for each problem.

Elimination

The data we have to support this problem is the patient's polyuria, which is a classic symptom of hyperglycemia. In addition, the patient is spilling glucose into his urine, also a classic sign of hyperglycemia. The patient's output is currently less than his input, which is likely to be a compensatory response by the body to the dehydrated state caused by polyuria. A review of the list of nursing diagnoses indicates that the diagnosis of *Impaired Urinary Elimination* is probably correct. To confirm the diagnosis, look up its definition, which says, "the state in which the individual experiences a disturbance in urine elimination."[19] This fits well with the data you have collected.

Nutrition

A patient with diabetes definitely has nutritional problems. This patient is on the 1800-calorie diabetic diet with no added sugar and is receiving insulin to regulate his blood glucose. A glucometer is being used regularly to monitor his blood glucose level, and his glycosylated hemoglobin level is elevated. In addition, the patient's cholesterol level is elevated, a problem that should be controlled to decrease his risk of coronary artery disease. The patient's records indicate that he had polydipsia and that currently his intake exceeds output, probably to compensate for the dehydration that occurred before he was regulated with replacement of insulin. The weakness is related to the starvation and dehydration that occurred without adequate insulin. Although the patient appears to be getting better, the diagnosis of *Imbalanced Nutrition: Less Than Body Requirements* is appropriate. It says, "the individual is experiencing an intake of nutrients insufficient to meet metabolic needs."[20]

Learning

All newly diagnosed patients need to learn about self-care. In this case, the patient needs to learn about the disease, how to prevent complications (as through foot care), medications such as insulin, the 1800 ADA diet, and exercise. Foot care and exercise would be added to the box that addresses patient learning needs. The appropriate diagnosis is *Deficient Knowledge*. The definition says, "absence or deficiency of cognitive information related to a specific topic."[21]

Anxiety

The patient said that he is anxious about learning to give himself injections and about following his diet. The diagnosis of *Anxiety* is defined as "a vague uneasy feeling of discomfort or dread accompanied by an autonomic response; the source is often nonspecific or unknown to the individual; a feeling of apprehension caused by anticipation of danger. It is an altering signal that warns of impending danger and enables the individual to take measures to deal with threat."[22] At this point, the patient appears to be a little anxious, probably because he does not know what is involved or if he will be capable of caring for himself.

Mobility

The patient has an increased risk of falling caused by weakness, and he is permitted to be OOB/chair. He can be diagnosed with *Impaired Physical Mobility,* which is defined as a "limitation in independent, purposeful physical movement of the body or of one or more extremities."[23]

BP Problems

The patient is receiving a BP medication and has a slightly elevated diastolic BP. Diabetes affects blood vessels all over the body, and most diabetic patients eventually develop cardiovascular and peripheral vascular disease. An appropriate nursing diagnosis is *Ineffective Tissue Perfusion (peripheral),* defined as "a decrease in oxygen resulting in the failure to nourish the tissues at the capillary level."[24] The patient will need instruction on slowing down the process of peripheral vascular complications, although these complications are inevitable. Peripheral vascular complications of diabetes affect circulation and sensation in the extremities, with skin breakdown and ulcerations as common consequences. Also, healing of wounds is much slower than normal with diabetes. It is clear now that the skin breakdown risk that you put in "I don't know how this fits with the problems" fits well with *Ineffective Tissue Perfusion.* Your map should now look like Figure 3.12.

Step 3: Mapping Cross-Links

Your concept care map is almost complete. Step 3 involves analyzing the relationships between the nursing diagnoses in order to make meaningful associations. The links must be accurate, meaningful, and complete. In concept care maps, the concepts you must link are the nursing diagnoses.

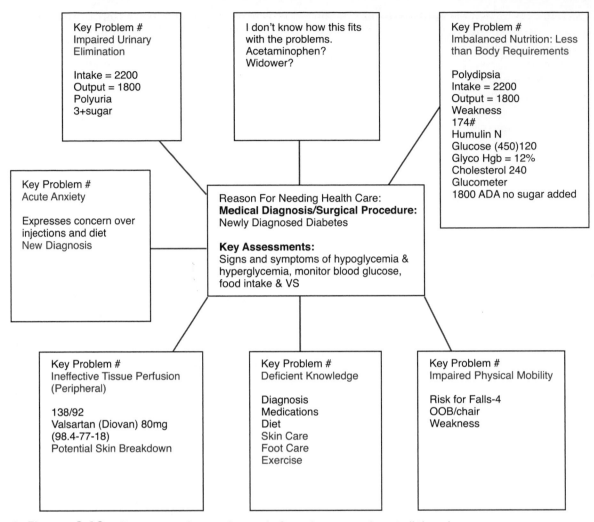

● Figure 3.12   Sloppy copy (preconference). Carry in your pocket at all times!

You must be able to state explicitly why you believe the diagnoses are related. Your faculty will be able to look at your map and see what was (or was not) in your mind and ask you questions about the relationships you indicated. So be prepared with good answers. The sloppy copy should now look like Figure 3.13.

Your explanations of the primary relationships between nursing diagnoses will be based on your knowledge of the disease process, as in the following examples.

▶ *Imbalanced Nutrition* and *Impaired Urinary Elimination:* These two concepts are always linked in any disease. What

goes in and is metabolized must come out in equal amounts, or there will be a health problem. Metabolism is altered with diabetes because a lack of insulin causes blood glucose to rise, and the excess glucose spills into the urine. As glucose is excreted, water is pulled out of the body by osmosis, creating an osmotic diuresis. Osmosis is the process by which a solution of higher concentration pulls water across a semipermeable membrane to equalize the concentrations on both sides of the membrane. Currently, the patient is making up for losses that created a state of dehydration by retaining

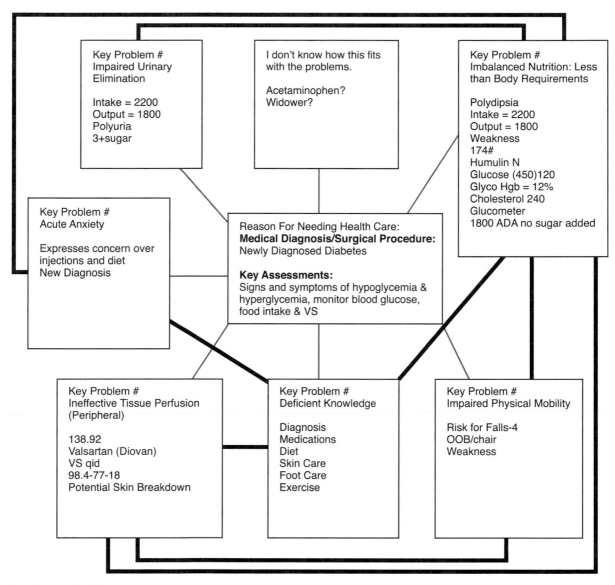

● Figure 3.13   Sloppy copy (preconference). Carry in your pocket at all times!

fluids. Thus, at this point, intake exceeds output.

▶ *Imbalanced Nutrition* and *Impaired Physical Mobility:* Without adequate nutrition, the body becomes weak and debilitated, leading to impaired physical mobility.

▶ *Imbalanced Nutrition* and *Ineffective Tissue Perfusion:* High blood glucose levels damage peripheral blood vessels, which in turn leads to problems with tissue oxygenation and nerve damage, leading to

hypertension, cardiovascular disease, peripheral neuropathies, nephropathies, foot ulcers, and infections.

▶ *Ineffective Tissue Perfusion* and *Impaired Physical Mobility:* Tissue perfusion problems, treatment with an antihypertensive, and neuropathies all influence a patient's mobility, giving him an increased risk of falling and an increased risk of skin breakdown.

▶ *Deficient Knowledge, Anxiety, Ineffective Tissue Perfusion,* and *Imbalanced*

Nutrition: Anxiety is common in newly diagnosed patients, no matter which health problem is involved. Anxiety may result from self-doubts about performing self-care and making lifestyle changes. Knowledge of the disease and treatments may serve to decrease patient anxiety. The patient must learn primarily about nursing diagnoses of nutrition and ineffective tissue perfusion. The patient will need to learn about the disease itself, including signs and symptoms, dietary management, blood glucose checks, insulin administration, exercise, and skin and foot care.

CHAPTER 3 SUMMARY

Important note: The diagnoses the night before clinical are primarily physiological and should always include anticipated knowledge deficits and psycho-social-emotional problems such as anxiety if you have the assessment data to support it. The focus of the initial plan is based only on data that are recorded and perhaps a brief introduction to your patient and a brief chat with the staff nurse.

Typically, little is formally written about the psycho-social-cultural assessment unless you are in a psychiatric setting. The psycho-social/cultural assessment is much less formal than the physiological assessment in most care settings, including home-care settings. You must spend time with the patient to do the psychosocial/cultural assessment; then you can add psycho-social-cultural diagnoses to the concept map on the day you care for the patient. This is the focus of Chapter 6.

The purpose of this chapter was to take you slowly through the first three steps of the concept care map planning process. After gathering clinical data, step 1 is to map the framework of propositions by noting the major medical diagnosis and the problems that result from that medical diagnosis. In step 2, organize the data into a hierarchy of subordinate concepts. This involves organizing abnormal physical assessment data, treatments, medications, diagnostic and laboratory tests, past medical problems, and emotional state under the problems listed in step 1. An important aspect of step 2 is the identification of key areas of assessment related to the primary medical diagnosis. Step 2 culminates in the final selection of nursing diagnoses based on the analysis of all available data. Step 3 involves the identification of meaningful associations between concepts on the map. The relationships between the nursing diagnoses are indicated with lines. The relationships you indicate must be accurate, meaningful, and complete; you should be prepared to explain why you believe a relationship exists between two connected diagnoses. In the Learning Activities, you will find two additional scenarios in Figures 3.14 and 3.15 that you can use to practice steps 1, 2, and 3 of the concept care mapping process.

LEARNING ACTIVITIES

1. Patient scenarios appear in Figures 3.14 and 3.15. Develop concept care maps for the data presented in these figures.

2. Compare concept care map diagrams with your classmates.

3. During class, explain to your classmates why you believe relationships exist between nursing diagnoses you have connected with lines in step 3.

Student Name: **MAB**

1) Date of Care: **12/24**	2) Patient Initials: **AL**	3) Age: **78** (face sheet)	3) Growth and Development **Ego integrity vs. Despair**	4) Gender: **F** (face sheet)	5) Admission Date: (face sheet) **12/3**

6) Reason for hospitalization (face sheet): Describe reason for hospitalization: (expand on back of page) *Medical Dx:* **Breast Cancer** *Pathophysiology:* *All signs and symptoms: Highlight those your patient exhibits*	7) Chronic illnesses (physician's history and physical notes in chart; nursing intake assessment and Kardex) **NIDDM** **Hypertension** **MI 1994**
8) Surgical procedures (consent forms and Kardex): Describe surgical procedure (expand on back of page) Name of surgical procedure: **Mastectomy** *Describe surgery:* **Right modified radical mastectomy**	

9) ADVANCE DIRECTIVES (NURSE'S ADMISSION ASSESSMENTS):

Living will: ☐ Yes ☐ No	Power of attorney: ☐ Yes ☐ No	Do not resuscitate (DNR) order (Kardex): ☐ Yes ☐ No

10) LABORATORY DATA:

Test	Normal Values	Admission 12/3	Date/Time 12/4	Date/Time	Reason for Abnormal Values
White blood cells (WBCs)		5.6	4.8		
Red blood cells (RBCs)					
Hemoglobin (Hgb)		11.2	11		
Hematocrit (Hct)		33.2	33.1		
Platelets		259,000			
Prothrombin time (PT)					
International normalized ratio (INR)					
Activated partial thromboplastin time (Aptt)					
Sodium Na					
Potassium K		2.8	2.8		
Chloride Cl					
Glucose (FBS/BS)		230	235		
Hemoglobin A1C					
Cholesterol					
Blood Urea Nitrogen (BUN)					
Creatinine					
Urine analysis (UA)					
Pre-albumin					
Albumin					
Calcium Ca					
Phosphate					
Bilirubin					
Alkaline phosphatase					
SGOT-Serum glutamic-oxyloacetic transaminase					
AST-Serum glutamic pyruvic transaminase					
CK					
CK MB					
Troponin					
B-natriuretic peptide BNP					
pH					
pCO_2					
pO_2					
HCO_3					

11) DIAGNOSTIC TESTS

Chest x-ray:	EKG:	Other abnormal reports:
Sputum or Blood Culture:	Other:	Other:

12) MEDICATIONS

List medications and times of administration (medication administration record and check the drawer in the carts for spelling). Include over-the-counter (OTC) products/herbal medicines

Times Due	1000	0800	1000	1000
Brand Name		Lasix	Tenormin	Zoloft
Generic Name	heparin	furosemide	atenolol	sertraline
Dose	5000U	40mg	25mg	25mg
Administration Route	sq	po	po	po
Classification				
Action				
Reason This Patient is Receiving				
Pharmacokinetics	O P D 1/2 M E	O P D 1/2 M E	O P D 1/2 M E	O P D 1/2 M E
Contraindications				
Major Adverse Side Effects				
Nursing Implications				
Pt/Family Teaching				

Developed by P. Testa, YSU

Times Due	1000	1000	1000	q4h pm
Brand Name	Lanoxin	Ecotrin	K-dur	Darvocet N-100
Generic Name	digoxin	aspirin	KCL	propoxyphene acetaminophen
Dose	01.25mg	1 tablet	20mg	100mg/650mg
Administration Route	po	po	po	po
Classification				
Action				
Reason This Patient is Receiving				
Pharmacokinetics	O P D 1/2 M E	O P D 1/2 M E	O P D 1/2 M E	O P D 1/2 M E
Contraindications				
Major Adverse Side Effects				
Nursing Implications				
Pt/Family Teaching				

Developed by P. Testa, YSU

ALLERGIES/PAINS

13) Allergies: **NKA** Type of Reaction: (medication administration record):	14) When was the last time pain medication given? (medication administration record) **Darvocet 6am (getting it sporadically)**
14) Where is the pain? **surgical incision** (nurse's notes)	14) How much pain is the patient in on a scale from 0-10? (nurse's notes, flow sheet): **5, confusion makes it unreliable**

TREATMENTS

15) List Treatments (Kardex): Rationale for treatments:
Dressing changes—sterile gauze & surgical bra, change qam
Ice to incision
Ted hose
IS q2h while awake
C&DB q2h while awake
I and O, & record q1h x 2

16) Support services (Kardex) What do support services provide for the patient?
17) What does the consultant do for the patient?:

18) DIET/FLUIDS

Type of Diet (Kardex): **1800 ADA**	Restrictions (Kardex):	Gag reflex intact: ☐ Yes ☐ No	Appetite: ☐ Good ☐ Fair ☒ Poor	Breakfast **Eating** **Jello and tea only**	Lunch _____ %	Dinner _____ %

What type of diet is this?:
What types of foods are included in this diet and what foods should be avoided?:

Circle Those Problems That Apply:	
Prior 24 hours Fluid intake: (Oral & IV) **2100** Fluid output **1700** (flow sheet)	• Problems: swallowing, chewing, dentures (nurse's notes) • Needs assistance with feeding (nurse's notes) • Nausea or vomiting (nurse's notes) • Overhydrated or dehydrated (evaluate total intake and output on flow sheet
Tube feedings: Type and rate (Kardex)	• Belching: • Other: _____ **Dentures and Needs Assistance Eating**

19) INTRAVENOUS FLUIDS (IV therapy record)

Type and Rate: **LR with 20 KCl 100/h**	IV dressing dry, no edema, redness of site: ☒ Yes ☐ No	Other:

20) ELIMINATION (flow sheet)

Last bowel movement: **None since surgery**	Foley/condom catheter: ☐ Yes ☒ No

Circle Those Problems That Apply:

• Bowel: constipation diarrhea flatus incontinence belching
• Urinary: hesitancy frequency burning incontinence odor
• Other: _____
• What is causing the problem in elimination? _____

21) ACTIVITY (Kardex, flow sheet)

Ability to walk (gait):	Type of activity orders: **up as tolerated**	Use of assistance devices: cane, walker, crutches, prosthesis:	Falls-risk assessment rating: **7 high**
No. of side rails required (flow sheet) **4**	Restraints (flow sheet): ☒ Yes ☐ No **vest, wrist**	Weakness ☒ Yes ☐ No	Trouble sleeping (nurse's notes): ☒ Yes ☐ No

What does activity order mean?: _____
Why isn't the patient up ad lib?: _____
Would the problem cause weakness?: _____

PHYSICAL ASSESSMENT DATA

22) BP (flow sheet): **137/72** **152/100**	2) TPR (flow sheet): **97-52-20** **97.8-80-20**	23) Height: __**5'5"**__ Weight: __**190#**__ (nursing intake assessments)

24) NEUROLOGICAL/MENTAL STATUS:

LOC: alert and oriented to person, place, time (A&O x 3), confused, etc. **Alert & oriented to person only, became confused evening after surgery**	Speech: clear, appropriate/inappropriate **inappropriate**
Pupils: PERRLA	Sensory deficits for vision/hearing/taste/ smell **glasses**

25) MUSCULOSKELETAL STATUS:

Bones, joints, muscles (fractures, contractures, arthritis, spinal curvatures, etc):	Extremity (temperature, edema (pitting vs. nonpitting) & sensation)
Motor: ROM x 4 extremities	
Ted hose/plexi pulses/compression devices: type:	Casts, splint, collar, brace:

26) CARDIOVASCULAR SYSTEM:

Pulses (radial, pedal) (to touch or with Doppler):	Capillary refill (<3s): ☐ Yes ☐ No	
Neck vein (distention):	Sounds: S1, S2, regular, irregular: Apical rate: **80**	Any chest pain:

27) RESPIRATORY SYSTEM:

Depth, rate, rhythm: **20**	Use of accessory muscles:	Cyanosis:	Sputum color, amount:	Cough: productive nonproductive	Breath sounds: clear, rales, wheezes **Clear, decreased in bases**
Use of oxygen: nasal cannula, mask, trach collar:	Flow rate of oxygen:	Oxygen humidification: ☐ Yes ☐ No		Pulse oximeter: _____ % oxygen saturation	Smoking: ☐ Yes ☐ No

28) GASTROINTESTINAL SYSTEM

Abdominal pain, tenderness, guarding; distention, soft, firm: **Soft & nondistended**	Bowel sounds x 4 quadrants: **Active 4 quads**	NG tube: describe drainage
Ostomy: describe stoma site and stools:	Other:	

29) SKIN AND WOUNDS:

Color, turgor: **Pink, poor turgor**	Rash, bruises: **Dry and chapped**	Describe wounds (size, locations): **Red & edematous**	Edges approximated: ☒ Yes ☐ No	Type of wound drains: **JP #1 25 ml** **JP #2 100 ml**
Characteristics of drainage: **serosanguineous**	Dressings (clean, dry, intact): **Clean, dry, intact**	Sutures, staples, steri-strips, other:	Risk for pressure ulcer assessment rating:	Other:

30) EYES, EARS, NOSE, THROAT (EENT):

Eyes: redness, drainage, edema, ptosis	Ears: drainage	Nose: redness, drainage, edema	Throat: sore

Psychosocial and Cultural Assessment

31) Religious preference (face sheet) **Catholic**	32) Marital status (face sheet) **Widowed**	33) Health care benefits and insurance (face sheet): **Medicare**
34) Occupation (face sheet) **Housewife**	35) Emotional state (nurse's notes) **Anxious, wants to go home, very talkative, does not respond to questions appropriately**	

● Figure 3.14   Patient profile database: Scenario 2—A surgical patient with a mastectomy.

Student Name: **BCD**

1) Date of Care: **2/5**	2) Patient Initials: **PUD**	3) Age: **55** (face sheet)	3) Growth and Development **Generativity vs. Stagnation**	4) Gender: **M** (face sheet)	5) Admission Date: (face sheet) **2/4**

6) Reason for hospitalization (face sheet): Describe reason for hospitalization: (expand on back of page) *Medical Dx:* **Arthritis, Chronic Pain right knee** *Pathophysiology:* *All signs and symptoms: Highlight those your patient exhibits*	7) Chronic illnesses (physician's history and physical notes in chart; nursing intake assessment and Kardex) **Hypertension**
8) Surgical procedures (consent forms and Kardex): Describe Surgical procedure (expand on back of page) Name of surgical procedure: **Right Knee Total Arthroplasty** *Describe surgery:*	

9) ADVANCE DIRECTIVES (NURSE'S ADMISSION ASSESSMENTS):

Living will: ☐ Yes ☐ No	Power of attorney: ☐ Yes ☐ No	Do not resuscitate (DNR) order (Kardex): ☐ Yes ☐ No

10) LABORATORY DATA:

Test	Normal Values	Admission 2/4	Date/Time	Date/Time	Reason for Abnormal Values
White blood cells (WBCs)		4.8			
Red blood cells (RBCs)					
Hemoglobin (Hgb)		12.5			
Hematocrit (Hct)		35.3			
Platelets		173,000			
Prothrombin time (PT)		11.5			
International normalized ratio (INR)					
Activated partial thromboplastin time (Aptt)		26.1			
Sodium Na					
Potassium K					
Chloride Cl					
Glucose (FBS/BS)					
Hemoglobin A1C					
Cholesterol					
Blood Urea Nitrogen (BUN)					
Creatinine					
Urine analysis (UA)					
Pre-albumin					
Albumin					
Calcium Ca					
Phosphate					
Bilirubin					
Alkaline phosphatase					
SGOT-Serum glutamic-oxyloacetic transaminase					
AST-Serum glutamic pyruvic transaminase					
CK					
CK MB					
Troponin					
B-natriuretic peptide BNP					
pH					
pCO_2					
pO_2					
HCO_3					

11) DIAGNOSTIC TESTS

Chest x-ray:	EKG:	Other abnormal reports:
Sputum or Blood Culture:	Other:	Other:

12) MEDICATIONS

List medications and times of administration (medication administration record and check the drawer in the carts for spelling). Include over-the-counter (OTC) products/herbal medicines.

Times Due	bid	qd	qd	q8h
Brand Name	K-dur	Hytrin	Colace	Kefzol
Generic Name	KCl	terazosin	docusate	cefazolin
Dose	20meq	5mg	100mg	1 g
Administration Route	po	po	po	po
Classification				
Action				
Reason This Patient is Receiving				
Pharmacokinetics	O P D 1/2 M E	O P D 1/2 M E	O P D 1/2 M E	O P D 1/2 M E
Contraindications				
Major Adverse Side Effects				
Nursing Implications				
Pt/Family Teaching				

Developed by P. Testa, YSU

Times Due	qd	q3-4h prn pain	q3-4h prn pain	q6h prn N?V
Brand Name	Lovenox	Demoral	Vicodin	Tigan
Generic Name	enoxaparin	meperidene	acetaminophen hydrocodone	trimethoben-zamid
Dose	30mg	75mg	500mg/5mg 1-2 tablets	200mg
Administration Route	sq	IM	po	IM
Classification				
Action				
Reason This Patient is Receiving				
Pharmacokinetics				
	O P D 1/2 M E	O P D 1/2 M E	O P D 1/2 M E	O P D 1/2 M E
Contraindications				
Major Adverse Side Effects				
Nursing Implications				
Pt/Family Teaching				

Developed by P. Testa, YSU

ALLERGIES/PAINS

13) Allergies: **sulfa, tetanus** Type of Reaction: (medication administration record):	14) When was the last time pain medication given? (medication administration record) **Darvocet 6am (getting it sporadically)**
14) Where is the pain? **incision** (nurse's notes)	14) How much pain is the patient in on a scale from 0-10? (nurse's notes, flow sheet): **8, decreased to 2 after meds**

TREATMENTS

15) List Treatments (Kardex): Rationale for treatments:

Dressing changes—begin po day 1
Ice to knee
Foley
IS q1h while awake with C&DB q2h while awake
CPM q shift for 3h

Mini-pillow under ankle
Plexi pulses
Overhead frame & trapeze

76

16) Support services (Kardex) What do support services provide for the patient?   **Physical Therapy to teach pt to use walker and CPM**

17) What does the consultant do for the patient?:

18) DIET/FLUIDS

Type of Diet (Kardex): **Regular**	Restrictions (Kardex):	Gag reflex intact: ☐ Yes ☐ No	Appetite: ☐ Good ☐ Fair ☐ Poor	Breakfast **75** %	Lunch **50** %	Dinner **75** %

What type of diet is this?:

What types of foods are included in this diet and what foods should be avoided?:

Circle Those Problems That Apply:	
Prior 24 hours Fluid intake: (Oral & IV) **1040** Fluid output **975** (flow sheet)	• Problems: swallowing, chewing, dentures (nurse's notes) • Needs assistance with feeding (nurse's notes) • Nausea or vomiting (nurse's notes) • Overhydrated or dehydrated (evaluate total intake and output on flow sheet
Tube feedings: Type and rate (Kardex)	• Belching: • Other: _____

19) INTRAVENOUS FLUIDS (IV therapy record)

Type and Rate: **Autotransfusion, D5W 1/2 NS 1000 ml q 12h**	IV dressing dry, no edema, redness of site: ☒ Yes ☐ No	Other:

20) ELIMINATION (flow sheet)

Last bowel movement: **2/3**	Foley/condom catheter: ☒ Yes ☐ No **clear yellow urine**

Circle Those Problems That Apply:

• Bowel: constipation diarrhea flatus incontinence belching
• Urinary: hesitancy frequency burning incontinence odor
• Other: _____
• What is causing the problem in elimination? _____

21) ACTIVITY (Kardex, flow sheet)

Ability to walk (gait): **Unsteady**	Type of activity orders: **WBAT**	Use of assistance devices: cane, walker, crutches, prosthesis: **Walker**	Falls-risk assessment rating: **5 high**
No. of side rails required (flow sheet) **2**	Restraints (flow sheet): ☐ Yes ☒ No	Weakness ☒ Yes ☐ No	Trouble sleeping (nurse's notes): ☐ Yes ☒ No

What does activity order mean?: _____
Why isn't the patient up ad lib?: _____
Would the problem cause weakness?: _____

PHYSICAL ASSESSMENT DATA

22) BP (flow sheet): **124/66**	2) TPR (flow sheet): **36.6**	23) Height: **5'11"** Weight: **202#** (nursing intake assessments)

24) NEUROLOGICAL/MENTAL STATUS:

LOC: alert and oriented to person, place, time (A&O x 3) confused, etc. **A&O x 3**	Speech: clear, appropriate/inappropriate **clear**
Pupils: **PERRLA**	Sensory deficits for vision/hearing/taste/ smell **glasses**

25) MUSCULOSKELETAL STATUS:

Bones, joints, muscles (fractures, contractures, arthritis, spinal curvatures, etc):	Extremity (temperature, edema (pitting vs. nonpitting) & sensation) **slight edema rt. Knee & lower leg**
Motor: ROM x 4 extremities **decreased rt. knee**	
Ted hose/plexi pulses/compression devices: type: **Plexi pulses on at all times while in bed**	Casts, splint, collar, brace:

26) CARDIOVASCULAR SYSTEM:

Pulses (radial, pedal) (to touch or with Doppler): **Pedals 3+ bilaterally**	Capillary refill (<3s): ☐ Yes ☐ No	
Neck vein (distention):	Sounds: S1, S2, regular, irregular: Apical rate:	Any chest pain:

27) RESPIRATORY SYSTEM:

Depth, rate, rhythm: **20**	Use of accessory muscles:	Cyanosis:	Sputum color, amount:	Cough: productive nonproductive	Breath sounds: clear, rales, wheezes **clear**
Use of oxygen: nasal cannula, mask, trach collar:	Flow rate of oxygen:	Oxygen humidification: ☐ Yes ☐ No		Pulse oximeter: ____ % oxygen saturation	Smoking: ☒ Yes ☐ No **history**

28) GASTROINTESTINAL SYSTEM

Abdominal pain, tenderness, guarding; distention, soft, firm: **Soft**	Bowel sounds x 4 quadrants: **+4 quads**	NG tube: describe drainage
Ostomy: describe stoma site and stools:	Other:	

29) SKIN AND WOUNDS:

Color, turgor:	Rash, bruises:	Describe wounds (size, locations): **Surgical incision bruised & edematous**	Edges approximated: ☒ Yes ☐ No	Type of wound drains: **Hemovac**
Characteristics of drainage: **Red 50cc**	Dressings (clean, dry, intact): **Clean, dry, intact**	Sutures, staples, steri-strips, other: **Sutures intact**	Risk for pressure ulcer assessment rating: **20 low risk**	Other:

30) EYES, EARS, NOSE, THROAT (EENT):

Eyes: redness, drainage, edema, ptosis	Ears: drainage	Nose: redness, drainage, edema	Throat: sore
Psychosocial and Cultural Assessment			
31) Religious preference (face sheet) **Presbyterian**	32) Marital status (face sheet) **Married**	33) Health care benefits and insurance (face sheet): **Aetna**	
34) Occupation (face sheet) **salesman**	35) Emotional state (nurse's notes) **calm, happy surgery is over**		

● Figure 3.15   Patient profile database: Scenario 3—A surgical patient with a knee replacement.

REFERENCES

1. Nursing's Social Policy Statement, ed 2. American Nurses Association, nursesbooks.org, Washington, D.C., 2003.
2. Novak, J, and Gowin, DB: Learning How to Learn. Cambridge University Press, New York, 1984 (reprinted 2002).
3. Ausubel, DP, et al: Educational Psychology: A Cognitive View, ed 2. Werbel and Peck, New York, 1986 (classic reference).

4. Deglin, JH, and Vallerand, AH: Davis's Drug Guide for Nurses: For PDA. FA Davis, Philadelphia, 2004.

5. Doenges, ME, et al: Nurse's Pocket Guide: Diagnoses, Interventions, and Rationales, ed 11. FA Davis, Philadelphia, 2008.

6. Ibid.

7. Brians, LK, et al: The development of the RISK tool for fall prevention. Rehabilitation Nursing 16(2):67, 1991.

8. Braden, B, and Bergstrom, N: In Bryant, RA (ed): Acute and Chronic Wounds: Nursing Management. Mosby, St. Louis, 1992.

9. NANDA Nursing Diagnoses: Definitions and Classification, 2007-2008. North American Nursing Diagnosis Association, Philadelphia, 2005.

10. Ibid.

11. Carpenito, LJ: Handbook of Nursing Diagnosis, ed 8. Lippincott, Philadelphia, 2005.

12. Ackley, BJ, and Ladwig, GB: Nursing Diagnosis Handbook, ed 6. Mosby, St. Louis, 2005.

13. Venes, D, et al. (eds): Taber's Cyclopedic Medical Dictionary, ed 20. FA Davis, Philadelphia, 2005.

14. Sparks, SM, and Taylor, CM: Nursing Diagnosis Reference Manual, ed 6. Springhouse, Springhouse, PA, 2004.

15. Gordon, M: Manual of Nursing Diagnosis, ed 11. Mosby, St. Louis, 2006.

16. Sparks, SM, and Taylor, CM: Op cit.

17. Gordon, M: Op cit.

18. NANDA: Op cit.

19. Ibid.

20. Ibid.

21. Ibid.

22. Ibid.

23. Ibid.

24. Ibid.

NURSING INTERVENTIONS:
So Many Problems, So Little Time

OBJECTIVES:

1. Identify the American Nurses Association (ANA) Standards of Clinical Nursing Practice related to identifying patient outcomes and planning nursing interventions.

2. Plan realistic and individualized goals, outcomes, and nursing interventions for each nursing diagnosis.

3. Include individualized physical and psychosocial interventions in each plan of care.

4. Develop an individualized teaching plan for the day of care.

5. Describe the use of information from standardized care plans to select typical interventions pertinent to the specific patient assignment on the day of care.

6. Recognize therapeutic communication techniques that will help to establish mutual goals, outcomes, and actions needed to ensure patient participation in health promotion, maintenance, and restoration.

The focus of this chapter is on step 4 of concept care mapping, which involves identifying therapeutic goals, outcomes, and nursing interventions and attaining patient and family participation in developing the care plan. The ANA Standards of Clinical Nursing Practice involving outcome identification and planning are standards 3, 4, and 5.[1] ANA standard 3 requires you to identify expected outcomes that must be individualized for your patient. For each nursing diagnosis, you must carefully identify the overall goal and specific patient outcomes. To do that, you need to know the progress that patients typically make in similar situations, and you need to know enough about the specifics of your patient's situation so you can accurately predict outcomes. Ask yourself, "What will this patient do on the day I'm assigned to care for her to demonstrate that she is making progress and moving toward a healthier state?" Often, patients have multiple problems, and such predictions may become difficult to make. Students commonly grow frustrated because a patient's condition changes between the time they gathered the patient data and the time they arrive on the unit to implement the plan of care. During the interlude, the patient's condition may have changed for better or worse, and the anticipated patient outcomes you created for the day will need to be revised. Sometimes, the patient may have been transferred or even discharged.

ANA standard 4 mandates that you are responsible for developing a plan of care that prescribes nursing interventions to attain the expected goals and outcomes. You must plan for the patient's physical and emotional care, and you must know what each intervention is intended to accomplish regarding the expected outcomes for the patient. In addition, your plan of care must include development of a specific teaching plan.

Therefore, one purpose of this chapter is to help you develop your critical thinking process in prioritizing problems, developing patient goals and outcomes, and selecting nursing interventions to attain those goals and outcomes. You will also work on developing a teaching plan for the diabetic patient introduced in earlier chapters.

In addition, this chapter will focus on gaining patient/family cooperation in the plan of care. It is important that you gain their cooperation by using therapeutic communication. The goals, expected outcomes, and activities to attain the goals and outcomes must be mutual. ANA standard 5 addresses the need for establishing mutual goals, outcomes, and interventions. This means that you must establish a therapeutic relationship so that the patient/family trusts you and is motivated to cooperate with the plan of care. Standard 5 specifies that the nursing actions must enable patient participation in all aspects of care, including health promotion, maintenance, and restoration. A therapeutic communication model is presented with special considerations given to gaining the cooperation of patients in establishing mutual goals, outcomes, and interventions.

Step 4: Thinking Critically About Patient Outcomes and Nursing Interventions

Review the concept care map shown in Figure 4.1. It is the one developed in Chapter 3 with a few details added. This concept care map diagram is prioritized and ready for use in the clinical setting. Note the patient's problem areas: nutrition, urinary elimination, mobility, anxiety, tissue perfusion, and knowledge deficits. It is important to be able to arrange these problem areas into priority order, to guide your nursing interventions as you deliver care to your patients and families.

Identifying Priority Problem No. 1

Find the box on the concept care map that has the most supporting data in it, and label it Problem No. 1. Usually, the most important diagnosis has the most supporting data and is the priority for planning care. In this example, *Imbalanced Nutrition* is the priority diagnosis. Given the pathophysiology of diabetes mellitus, it makes sense that the patient's nutritional state is going to be highly disrupted, and the patient will need interventions to promote healthy nutrition. Now, for this problem, you will assign outcomes; think critically to determine nursing interventions; and document the problems, goals, outcomes, and interventions.

Assigning Outcomes

As a general goal, the patient would be expected to continue improving his nutritional status. It is important to assess the patient's progress toward this goal and to discern what needs to be accomplished to achieve a healthier state.

For this particular patient, the last known blood glucose level was at 110 mg/dL. Normal blood glucose levels are 80 to 110 mg/dL. Therefore, a major predicted outcome is that the patient will maintain his blood sugar between 80 mg/dL and 110 mg/dL by eating his 1800-calorie diet and taking insulin injections as scheduled.

Nursing Interventions

What must you do to make sure the patient attains this outcome? Use the box of patient data

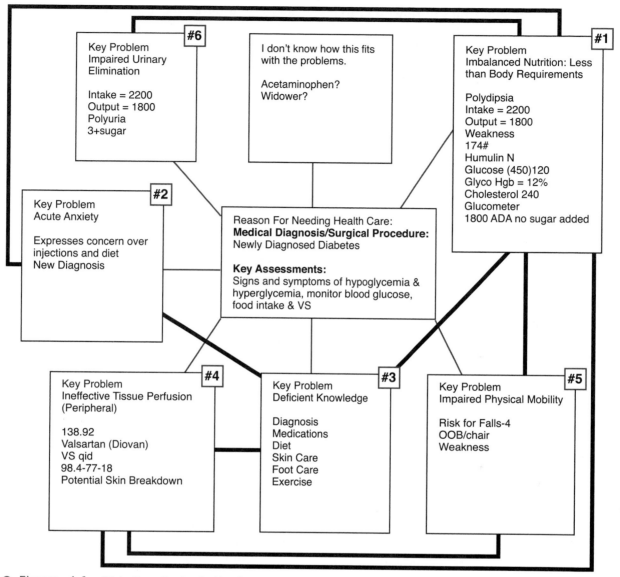

● Figure 4.1   Diabetic patient-prioritized problems.

you diagnosed as *Imbalanced Nutrition*. The box of data on your concept care map gives many clues as to what your interventions will involve:

▶ Assess the abdomen.
▶ Assess the patient for hyperglycemia, and obtain a medication order to give additional insulin if indicated.
▶ Assess the patient's blood glucose with the glucometer.
▶ Monitor the patient's appetite, and encourage the patient to eat his meals.
▶ Administer his insulin injections as scheduled.

▶ Watch for signs and symptoms of hypoglycemia, especially if the patient's intake is not sufficient.

Continuous assessment is the first priority for each nursing intervention list. It is critically imperative to focus on the primary system of the body affected; in this case, the gastrointestinal (GI) system. Therefore, the first intervention that should be listed is always the assessment you intend to perform to monitor the physical signs and symptoms of the nursing diagnosis. The basic GI assessment includes bowel sounds, abdominal tenderness, distention, and bowel movements.

Assessments include monitoring for hypoglycemia and hyperglycemia.

Take another look at the data in the box for nutrition. What about the polydipsia and 2200-cc intake and 1800-cc output? Continue to monitor the patient's intake and output. Remember that polydipsia and polyuria are classic signs of hyperglycemia, and this patient became dehydrated before he was hospitalized. Currently, his intake exceeds his output because his body is trying to make up for the fluid losses.

The patient's weakness stems from lack of food and from dehydration. Therefore, monitor his appetite and encourage him to consume his 1800-calorie diet, no sugar added. Calories and food types must be regulated carefully against the amount of insulin administered and the patient's level of exercise. Usually, it takes several days of blood glucose monitoring and insulin adjustment before a patient's daily diet, exercise, and insulin patterns can be stabilized. In regulating diabetic patients, it is imperative that there be a counterbalance among calories consumed, insulin dosages, and exercise.

Keep in mind that this patient's weakness is a safety risk. Caution is warranted when transferring him and helping him ambulate. As he continues to progress, he should become stronger. Assess his weakness level when you first meet him on the day of care by asking him how much help he needs walking. His risk for falls may also be partly related to his antihypertensive therapy and his age. Antihypertensive drugs commonly cause orthostatic hypotension, which is a drop in blood pressure that causes symptoms of lightheadedness when the patient changes positions, particularly when moved from lying down to sitting or standing up. As people age, the valves inside veins commonly weaken, which can encourage pooling of blood in the periphery and which also may result in orthostatic hypotension. To determine the possible effects of orthostatic hypotension on your patient, check his blood pressure and pulse while he sits on the side of his bed. Also, before you help him stand up, ask him whether he gets dizzy when he stands up. That way, you will reduce the patient's risk of falling and possibly becoming injured.

The rest of the data in the nutrition box on your concept care map addresses additional blood work to check glycohemoglobin (Hgb A_{1c})

and cholesterol. Blood samples would not be drawn every day. You must plan to check the results of any blood work that is ordered, however, and to promptly report abnormal values to your clinical faculty and the patient's doctor. For example, the doctor may have ordered that electrolytes be drawn. Review those reports as soon as they become available. Always be aware of the time that any blood work is done and the time the reports should be available. Sometimes, blood samples get lost. If the reports are not available as scheduled, you may need to contact the laboratory to make sure the blood sample was received and is being processed.

Writing Problems, Goals, Objectives, Outcomes, and Interventions

A blank sample format to guide you in writing out problems, goals, objectives, outcomes, and interventions is shown in Figure 4.2. Figure 4.3 contains goals, objectives, outcomes, and interventions for this diabetic patient scenario. You have identified nutrition as the top priority for your patient, so write it as Problem No. 1, and list the goals and expected outcomes under this problem. Under the column labeled "Nursing Interventions," write brief notes of all the things you are planning to do, based on what you believe to be important from your analysis of the information in the nutrition box. The right-hand column on the form is reserved for direct observations made of the patient during the clinical day. You will record the patient's responses to each intervention and thus use this column to evaluate the patient. This process is explained further in Chapter 5.

The interventions listed so far can be classified as physically supportive of the patient. Nurses perform physical assessments (GI system), use equipment to monitor patients (glucometer), monitor laboratory and diagnostic tests (blood glucose), administer medications (insulin), and perform treatments (none for this particular diagnosis).

Identifying Priority Problem No. 2

Look at the concept care map again. *Anxiety* and *Knowledge Deficits* are very important interacting diagnoses. Recall that there is a direct line

Problem #_____ :
General Goal:

Predicted Behavioral Outcome Objective (s): The patient will...
_____
_____
_____on the day of care.

Nursing Interventions	Patient Responses to Interventions
1._____	1._____
2._____	2._____
3._____	3._____
4._____	4._____
5._____	5._____
6._____	6._____
7._____	7._____
8._____	8._____

Evaluation: Summarize patient progress toward outcome objectives:
_____
_____

Problem #_____ :
General Goal:

Predicted Behavioral Outcome Objective (s): The patient will...
_____
_____
_____on the day of care.

Nursing Interventions	Patient Responses to Interventions
1._____	1._____
2._____	2._____
3._____	3._____
4._____	4._____
5._____	5._____
6._____	6._____
7._____	7._____
8._____	8._____

Evaluation: Summarize patient progress toward outcome objectives:
_____
_____

● Figure 4.2 Format for writing problems, goals, objectives, interventions, and responses, and summary.

drawn between Acute Anxiety and Deficient Knowledge, indicating the relationship between these nursing diagnoses. The goals are to decrease anxiety and increase knowledge of diabetes. When anxiety is decreased, the patient will be able to learn better, and when he has knowledge of self-care, he will have less anxiety about his ability to perform self-care. Anxiety is a common emotional reaction to the stress of illness. For this patient, anxiety may result from his recognition that he must make changes in his lifestyle and that he lacks the confidence and

Problem #__1__: Imbalanced Nutrition: Less than body requirements
General Goal: To improve the patient's nutritional status

Predicted Behavioral Outcome Objective (s): The patient will…maintain his blood glucose between 80 and 120 mg/dl by eating his 1800-calorie ADA diet and administering insulin injections as scheduled… on the day of care.

Nursing Interventions	Patient Responses to Interventions
1. Assess abdomen: bowel sounds, tenderness, distention, BMs	1.
2. Assess blood glucose with glucometer at 0800 and 1100	2.
3. Assess S/S of hypoglycemia and hyperglycemia	3.
4. Monitor appetite—1800 cal ADA, no sugar added	4.
5. Measure fluid intake and output	5.
6. Administer insulin on time	6.
7. Check for additional blood work	7.
8. Monitor patient for orthostatic hypotension and weakness	8.
9. Ambulate carefully to avoid falls	9.

● Figure 4.3   Problem No. 1.

knowledge to make those changes. Consequently, his anxiety must be assessed and reduced before teaching will be successful.

Therefore, anxiety reduction takes priority over patient education. Label it priority Problem No. 2 on your map (Fig. 4.4). Patients are not able to concentrate and learn when anxiety is high. The net result of too much anxiety is usually impaired cognitive function, which simply means that the brain does not work as well.

Short-term memory, concentration, and abstract thought can be altered in high-anxiety states. Patients' thoughts are blocked; patients may appear confused and forgetful; and they may have difficulty concentrating. All of these factors contribute to a decreased learning ability. A little anxiety, however, can be motivational. If the patient is slightly anxious, his senses are on full alert, and he can use the increased alertness and energy to his advantage to learn about self-care.

Problem #__2__: Anxiety
General Goal: Decrease Anxiety

Predicted Behavioral Outcome Objective (s): The patient will…verbalize concerns about his disease and the changes that must be made in his lifestyle… on the day of care.

Nursing Interventions	Patient Responses to Interventions
1. Assess current level of anxiety	1.
2. Use empathy	2.
3. Use therapeutic touch	3.
4. Use therapeutic humor	4.

● Figure 4.4   Problem No. 2.

The goal is to decrease the patient's anxiety but not to completely obliterate it.

The outcome for an anxious patient is to verbalize concerns and express himself. The appropriate interventions include therapeutic communication techniques to facilitate ventilation of feelings and thus relieve anxiety. The first intervention listed is to assess anxiety (remember, assessment first), then attempt therapeutic communication techniques such as empathy, therapeutic touch, and therapeutic use of humor to reduce anxiety in this patient situation. What do you say to someone who is anxious to help them reduce their anxiety? How do you know that someone is anxious?

Once you believe the problem is anxiety, use a basic care planning book to confirm the diagnosis. Look up the nursing diagnosis *Anxiety* and see the defining characteristics to determine the behavioral, affective, physiological, and cognitive defining characteristics of anxiety. For example, a partial list from NANDA for the defining characteristics of anxiety includes insomnia, fidgeting, poor eye contact, and restlessness. Some affective signs of anxiety include irritability, uncertainty, and feelings of inadequacy. Physiological signs include facial tension, increased heart rate, and blood pressure. Cognitive signs include forgetfulness and impaired attention. In the NANDA reference, there are 69 listed defining characteristics for anxiety that should be assessed. If you assess each of the 69 characteristics of anxiety, you almost always find a patient will be displaying some of these signs. In working with every patient, always assess anxiety. Anxiety results in painful emotions that always accompany physical and mental illness.

Therapeutic Communication

Nurses must be able to determine psychosocial and emotional effects of health problems such as anxiety. Nurses need to learn therapeutic communication techniques to assess psychosocial and emotional effects of the health problem. In developing a plan of care to be emotionally supportive to patients, there are therapeutic communication techniques that every nurse should integrate into every plan of care. What are communication interventions nurses use to give emotional support to patients? These are briefly reviewed below.

Empathy is a very important communication technique to learn for dealing with patients' painful emotional responses. The classic emotions of sadness, fear, and anger are prevalent during illness. Without release, emotional feelings of sadness can progress to clinical depression; specific fears can progress to diffuse anxiety; and anger may be manifested as hostility and resentment.

Allow the patient to have an emotional release by acknowledging and accepting his emotions and by encouraging him to express those emotions. Do not pretend that his emotions do not exist. Do not criticize emotions. Do not try to rationalize emotions. Do not try to change or fix emotions. At first, the person may yell or blame. He may placate and cry. Or he may be sarcastic and make jokes about his problems. After this period of ventilation, however, he may be able to express his frustrations with his current situation and begin to problem-solve.

Therapeutic touch can be used to decrease the patient's response to anxiety. Carefully monitor the patient's responses to touch. Touch needs to be related to the context of the situation. *Caring touch* includes holding the patient's hand, placing an arm around his shoulders, giving him a hug or a pat on the back. Touch can be used to support, reassure, and raise spirits. *Protective touch* is used where patient safety is a primary concern. A confused patient may be restrained and sedated to make sure he will not pull on vital tubes or fall out of bed. When applying restraints, use caring touch at the same time. *Task touch* involves physical assessment and procedural treatments that must be done. Be gentle and careful with task touches, and overlap them with caring touches.

Therapeutic humor addresses situational dilemmas or points out human weaknesses. Sometimes humor can help to reduce mild anxiety and put people at ease. When people can see the absurdity in a situation and laugh at it, they can distance themselves from threatening problems. Humor is an effective coping mechanism that helps to reframe reality and reduce negative feelings. It facilitates the experience of relief from painful emotions. It is important not to be insulting when using humor and to assess the patient carefully for physical and emotional discomforts before using therapeutic humor. Therapeutic communication interventions are shown in Box 4.1. In addition to the physical care of patients, nurses focus on emotional support and specific communication interventions of empathy, touch, and humor.

Learning how to gain the cooperation and respect of patients when you are a "rookie" nursing student is covered in detail in Schuster's *Communication: The Key to the Therapeutic Relationship.*[2] A summary of what you must know to communicate effectively and develop therapeutic communication skills is included in Box 4.2.

| Box 4.1 | THERAPEUTIC COMMUNICATION TECHNIQUES |

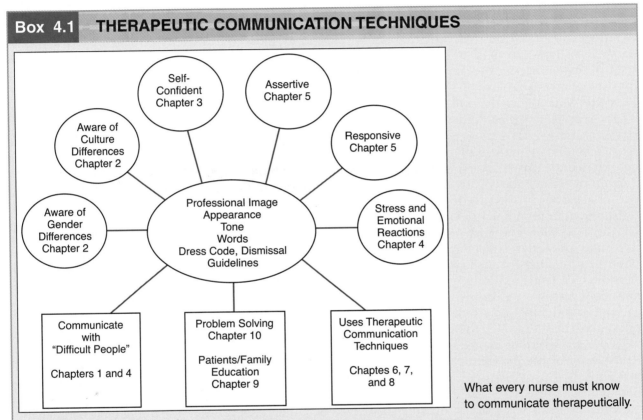

What every nurse must know to communicate therapeutically.

Expressions of Sadness and Grief

Tears and crying are very important therapeutic resources that can be used to facilitate healing and well-being. Tears are a natural way of releasing tension that comes from sadness, grief, anger, and fear. Nursing a patient with a loss involves allowing the patient to experience an emotional release through tears. Avoid expressing disapproval or minimizing the cause of crying, and do not offer false hope or make promises that you cannot keep to make the crying stop. Listen supportively and empathetically to patient and family verbalizations of emotional pain.

Building Self-Esteem

Self-esteem is the value a person places on himself and affects the way he interacts with others. Health problems commonly lower self-esteem. Those patients with low self-esteem may have feelings of isolation, helplessness, incompetence, or being unloved. To build self-esteem, define clear and realistic goals, help patients think clearly, give positive feedback, encourage positive self-affirmations, and use visualization exercises.

Anticipatory Guidance

Nurses use anticipatory guidance to guide patients through uncomfortable procedures. Talk to your patients, and explain the sensations they will be feeling so they know what to expect, and their anxiety will be reduced. For example, when giving an intramuscular injection, say something like, "First I'll palpate and find the right spot. Then you will feel me wiping you off. Then you will feel a pinch and a little burning. It's the medication....All done. I'm massaging the site a little."

Reminiscing and Life Review

When using reminiscing, the nurse encourages the patient to recall and talk about life experiences. Reminiscing can be helpful in resocializing people and building relationships, whereas the life review helps people make sense of their lives and see their lives as unique stories. Nurses implement reminiscence or life review to help patients deal with crises and losses, to prevent and reduce depression, and to increase life satisfaction.

Distraction

Distraction is a technique used to take a patient's mind off what is bothering her. The patient may be waiting nervously for a procedure. She is prepared for it as well as can be, so you make small talk about whatever interests her. This distraction also works when you are trying to get a slightly confused patient to cooperate with you. For example, you have a slightly confused elderly patient who is demanding to go for a walk right now, despite having a nasogastric tube, catheters, and intravenous lines. Although you may need to use light restraints, you may also be able to distract the person from her demand by getting her interested in the television, a magazine, or a conversation.

Problem Solving and Decision Making

Nurses commonly help patients solve problems and make decisions. The steps of the problem-solving or decision-making process include identifying the problem, searching for information about the problem, identifying options, examining the pros and cons of each option, choosing an option, developing a plan of action, implementing the plan, and evaluating the effects.

Schuster, P. Communication: The Key to the Therapeutic Relationship. FA Davis, Philadelphia, 2000.

Identifying Priority Problem No. 3

The third priority problem for this patient is deficient knowledge of self-care. Label it as Problem No. 3 on your concept map. It is a nursing responsibility to educate each patient about self-care and to include significant others in the teaching. According to data you have collected for your concept care map, this patient is most concerned about injections and diet. One of your first interventions may be to assess his knowledge of injections, diet, and other self-care activities (Fig. 4.5). Also ask your patient's staff nurse what information she has attempted to teach him and how he has responded to teaching.

As you collected patient data, there was no mention in the patient's records that he had seen a diabetes educator or had attended classes. Find out what resources are available to bridge the gap between what he knows and what he needs to learn. Check to see what types of classes are available to the patient, whether the dietitian has been to talk to him, and whether a diabetes educator is available.

Each patient (and significant other) needs a teaching plan centered on the day of care. This diabetic patient needs to know about his diagnosis, medications, diet, exercise, and skin care. He cannot possibly learn all of that in one day, but you must develop a general teaching plan before meeting with the patient.

Box 4.2   HOW TO BECOME A THERAPEUTIC COMMUNICATOR

Objective 1: Recognize current communication patterns:

1. General assessment: How well do you communicate? (Chapter 1)
2. Gender differences in communication (Chapter 2): Male and female patterns of communication—sex talk quiz, brain sex test
3. Cultural differences in communication (Chapter 2): Communication in families (touch, punctuality, ethnicity, family—mini cultural assessment; touch avoidance scale)
4. Self-confidence (Chapter 3): Self-esteem, body image; making a positive impression (How Do You See Yourself Scale)
5. Assertiveness (Chapter 5): Willing to take a stand; able to defend beliefs; independent/forceful/ dominant/leader (assessing assertiveness; communication competence scale)
6. Responsive (Chapter 5): Sensitive to needs of others; attentive listener; desire to make others feel at ease (communication competence scale)

Objective 2: Analyze how to establish trust and rapport in nurse-patient relationships

1. Recognizing common patterns of communication behaviors when the patient is under stress: "Difficult" communication situations (Chapters 1 and 4): Blamers, placators, computers, distractors, levelers (aggressive/angry: openly hostile, slurs, insults, sarcasm; passive: too agreeable, "says yes, means no," procrastinating; complaining)
2. Dealing with difficult people using therapeutic communication techniques: Empathy (Chapters 1 and 4): recognizes/reads emotions person is expressing under stress, verbally responds to the emotion (comments on the emotion); asks the patient to verbalize the underlying problem; uses problem solving or refers problem: how to respond to hostility, sarcasm, procrastinators, complaining; Touch (Chapter 6); Humor (Chapter 7); Interventions with tears (Chapter 8); Patient education (Chapter 9)
3. Assisting patients to analyze a problem and assisting them in decision making (Chapter 10): identification of problems, steps in problem solving and decision making (examples: Management of Self-Care Deficits at Home and Caregiver Role Strain)

To determine the content of your teaching plan, review a standardized nursing care plan book or software program for educating patients about major diseases. While obtaining your patient assignment at the health-care agency, get any available teaching aids about his health problems. Read them carefully so you understand the basics of what the patient needs to know. From these resources, pick out the essential teaching information pertinent to your patient.

Identifying Priority Problem No. 4

Review your concept care map, and look at the remaining diagnoses to select the problem of the fourth priority. The box with the diagnosis *Ineffective Tissue Perfusion (Peripheral)* contains more patient profile data than the boxes with impaired mobility or impaired elimination, so you can label it Problem No. 4. The pathophysiology of diabetes affects the circulation; many diabetics have a history of hypertension. Specifically, diabetes speeds up degeneration of the arteries and veins, and fat deposits build up in the blood vessels, leading to atherosclerosis and hypertension. Atherosclerosis is the cause of coronary artery disease (heart attacks), cerebral vascular disease (strokes), and peripheral vascular disease (ulcers). Peripheral vascular disease has many implications for diabetics. With inade-

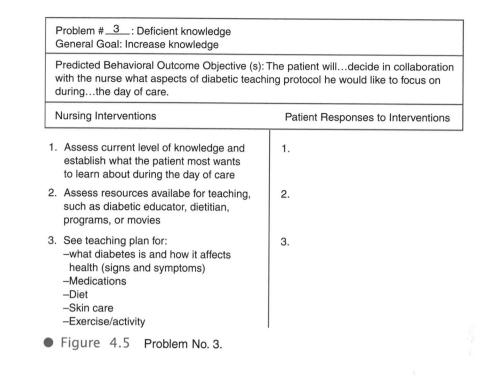

Problem #__3__: Deficient knowledge
General Goal: Increase knowledge

Predicted Behavioral Outcome Objective (s): The patient will…decide in collaboration with the nurse what aspects of diabetic teaching protocol he would like to focus on during…the day of care.

Nursing Interventions	Patient Responses to Interventions
1. Assess current level of knowledge and establish what the patient most wants to learn about during the day of care	1.
2. Assess resources availabe for teaching, such as diabetic educator, dietitian, programs, or movies	2.
3. See teaching plan for: –what diabetes is and how it affects health (signs and symptoms) –Medications –Diet –Skin care –Exercise/activity	3.

● Figure 4.5   Problem No. 3.

quate tissue perfusion, tissues will break down, and pressure ulcers will form. Nerve degeneration also occurs in the periphery. This is termed *diabetic neuropathy* and results in pain, tingling, and burning in the legs. Neuropathy progresses to a lack of sensation in the legs as the disease worsens.

Therefore, the general goal is to maintain optimal tissue perfusion and circulation (Fig. 4.6). Specific outcomes include keeping the patient's vital signs close to normal and avoiding skin breakdown. The first intervention is always assessment. You will assess his vital signs and will assess his circulation by checking capillary refill and peripheral pulses. You will also assess for skin breakdown and pressure ulcers. Other interventions include encouraging supervised ambulation, helping the patient into a chair, and encouraging the patient to perform range-of-motion exercises to improve circulation to his limbs and prevent skin breakdown.

Identifying Priority Problems Nos. 5 and 6

The two remaining diagnoses that have not been directly addressed include *Impaired Physical Mobility* and *Impaired Urinary Elimination*. These diagnoses are of equal importance and have been labeled Problems No. 5 and No. 6 on the concept care map. It does not matter which is Problem No. 5 and which is Problem No. 6, as long as both are recognized as problems.

The goal for *Impaired Physical Mobility* is to prevent complications of immobility and to prevent falls. The patient outcomes are to sit in a chair with assistance, to perform range-of-motion exercises, and to ambulate as much as tolerated. Interventions to attain these outcomes have been covered in Problem Nos. 1 and 4. Specifically, you will monitor the patient for orthostatic hypotension and weakness, and you will carefully assist the patient with ambulation to avoid falls. You will also help the patient sit in a chair and perform range-of-motion exercises.

The goal for *Impaired Urinary Elimination* is to maintain normal urinary elimination. Outcomes include intake and output approaching normal values and the patient having no polyuria. Interventions are covered under Problem No. 1 and include measuring fluid intake and output and monitoring for signs and symptoms of hyperglycemia and hypoglycemia.

The goals and outcomes for *Impaired Physical Mobility* and *Impaired Urinary Elimination*

Problem #__4__ : Ineffective Tissue Perfusion (peripheral)
General Goal: Maintain optimal tissue perfusion and circulation

Predicted Behavioral Outcome Objective (s): The patient will...have vital signs remaining close to normal, no skin breakdown, moves safely from bed to chair...on the day of care.

Nursing Interventions	Patient Responses to Interventions
1. Assess vital signs	1.
2. Assess peripheral pulses and capillary refill	2.
3. Assess skin for pressure sore	3.
4. Give valsartan, assess BP/P prior to administrations	4.
5. ROM extremities q2h if in bed	5.
6. Walk w/assistance	6.
7. Chair x 2	7.

● Figure 4.6   Problem No. 4.

are shown in Figure 4.7. There is no need to copy interventions that you have already specified into this summary. Instead, refer to the interventions covered under previous nursing diagnoses.

Your basic care map is now complete with goals, objectives, outcomes, and interventions. You can carry the concept care map, complete with goals, outcomes, interventions, and teaching plan, in your pocket on the clinical units and use it during the implementation phase of the nursing process. Be prepared to discuss with your clinical faculty the rationales for each of the interventions you identified. Although the basic care map is complete, you still need to develop a teaching plan. What follows is a discussion of one method for developing a teaching plan.

Problem #__5__ : Impaired Physical Mobility
General Goal: Prevent complications of immobility, prevent falls

Predicted Behavioral Outcome Objective (s): The patient will...ambulate to chair and walk with steady gait, does range of motion exercises...on the day of care.

Nursing Interventions	Patient Responses to Interventions
1. Covered under Nutrition and Altered tissue perfusion	

Problem #__6__ : Impaired Urinary Elimination
General Goal: Maintain normal urinary elimination

Predicted Behavioral Outcome Objective (s): The patient will...have intake and output approaching normal values, no polyuria...on the day of care.

Nursing Interventions	Patient Responses to Interventions
1. Covered under Nutrition	

● Figure 4.7   Problem Nos. 5 and 6.

Developing a Mini–Teaching Plan Using METHOD

Development of a one-page mini–individualized teaching plan with specific content and teaching methods is the focus of the last section of this chapter. Box 4.3 shows an outline that you can use to develop a one-page mini–teaching plan. This outline focuses on key information that all patients and significant others need to know about their specific disease and its treatments. The key teaching areas are structured around the acronym METHOD.[3,4]

Using a specific method to teach content (in this case, the acronym) will help you remember key items to cover in every teaching plan you construct. Teaching is an essential component of all care planning. Students are required to come to clinical prepared to teach whatever is appropriate for the clinical day. If you are assigned to a preoperative patient, focus on preoperative teaching. If you are assigned to a first-day surgical patient, focus teaching on the first day after surgery. Focus on discharge teaching if the patient is being prepared to go home while you are taking care of him.

M is for Medications

Write the name (generic and brand name) and key action for each drug. Write one sentence for each drug that represents how you would explain it to your patient in words the patient and his significant others can understand. Avoid using medical terminology from your drug guides. Use medical terminology only when explaining a drug's actions and side effects to your clinical faculty as you are preparing the drugs for administration. For example, write:

- ▶ "This is an antibiotic for your infection."
- ▶ "This is a blood thinner to prevent clots."
- ▶ "This is your pain pill."
- ▶ "This is your insulin to control your blood sugar."

Details about side effects are not necessary unless the patient is going home with the drug or is asking for more specific information. If he is going home with the drug, write the basics of what you will say in simple terms with as few words as possible. For example, "Take Tylenol (acetaminophen) if you need something for discomfort. Don't take aspirin because it is a blood thinner." or "Take your antibiotic three times a day: when you get up, in the afternoon, and at night before bed. Take the entire prescription. Don't stop before it's finished, even if you feel better. Take it with food if your stomach gets upset." Write down information if the patient is being discharged so he will have reminders when he is home what is to be done and why.

E is for Environment

Environment includes home or health-care agency environment, financial considerations, and social support. Review standardized nursing care plan guides and nursing texts to determine how the patient and his significant others may need to modify the home environment. Assess the patient's home situation, and intervene if needed. Determine whether the patient has the financial resources to implement the treatment plan, and intervene if necessary. Find out whether the patient has significant others to assist with care if needed. If significant others are not available, contacts with community agencies may be necessary to assist in the adjustment to returning home. Also consider what you must do to provide a safe environment in the health-care setting. For example, does the patient need furniture arranged so he may safely get up to a chair or walk to the bathroom? Is the call light in reach, is the bed down, are the side rails up, and are the wheels locked on the patient's bed? Patients and family members must be taught how to arrange their environments to prevent accidents.

T is for Treatments

Explain the purpose of each treatment and the correct techniques for performing treatments that will continue at home. For example, explain skin care procedures or wound care. Write down specifically what the patient needs to do. If written guidelines are available, highlight the most important things for the patient to remember. Exercise or activity guidelines may also be con-

Box 4.3	METHOD DAILY TEACHING PLAN

Patient name:

Diagnosis:

Teaching techniques:

M (Medications):

_____

_____

_____

_____

E (Environment):

_____

_____

_____

T (Treatment):

_____

_____

_____

_____

H (Health Knowledge of Disease):

_____

_____

_____

_____

O (Outpatient/Inpatient Referrals):

_____

_____

_____

_____

D (Diet):

_____

_____

_____

_____

sidered a treatment. Each patient must be aware of activities that are and are not permitted and how to develop and maintain an exercise routine. Many diabetic patients will be instructed to increase their walking gradually until they are walking for 30 minutes every day.

H is for Health Knowledge of Disease

Write down the effects of the patient's disease, signs and symptoms that he should watch for, and any changes that should prompt him to call the physician or nurse practitioner. For example, write down what the patient should watch for regarding signs and symptoms of an infection in a wound, a urine infection, or whatever is applicable to the specific patient problems.

O is for Outpatient/Inpatient Referrals

Write a sentence to explain inpatient diagnostic tests or procedures using nonmedical terms. For outpatient referrals, list support groups, home health agencies, office appointments, and any pertinent dates and times. Check with the staff nurse assigned to your patient during your assigned clinical day to find out the physician's usual routine for patients after discharge. Also, read the discharge orders.

D is for Diet

Write down the patient's appropriate diet and restrictions. Obtain examples of typical menus from the dietitian. Write down a list of foods that the patient can eat and foods that he should avoid as applicable.

Sample METHOD Plan for a Diabetic Patient

For your diabetic patient, the METHOD teaching plan will result from a synthesis of concept care map data, standardized teaching plans, and patient education materials for diabetic patients. You will need to review a standardized teaching plan for diabetics, standardized insulin patient information, standardized 1800-calorie American Diabetes Association (ADA) diet samples, and patient education booklets on diabetes. The following section walks you through the construction of a METHOD teaching plan for this patient.

Medications

Three drugs are listed on your concept care map: humulin N, valsartan, and acetaminophen. Based on information you glean from drug references, your patient teaching information about the patient's medications may look like Box 4.4. It is formatted using the actual words you might say to the patient. Keep in mind that although this section of the teaching plan is written to the patient, the plan is for your use, not to be given to the patient. Naturally, you should be prepared to discuss the details of your teaching plan with your clinical faculty before giving a drug or even giving the patient this information. You should also be prepared to give the patient more information if he asks for it.

Environment

Your patient is an 80-year-old widower. He has insurance. To fill out this section of the teaching

---

Box 4.4   METHOD DAILY TEACHING PLAN

Patient Name: ET
Diagnosis: Newly diagnosed diabetes
Teaching techniques: Give explanations, one-on-one discussion, demonstrations
M (Medications): Humulin N (NPH, human insulin) insulin: "This drug is to control blood glucose levels. Watch for signs and symptoms of hypoglycemia and hyperglycemia. Onset (1 to 2 hours), peak (6 to 12 hours), and duration (up to 24 hours). Take this drug each morning 30 minutes before breakfast. If you do not eat as scheduled and in the amounts specified in your diet plan, you will

probably have a hypoglycemic reaction in mid to late afternoon (6 to 12 hours after you've taken the drug)."
Valsartan (Diovan): "This drug is to control your blood pressure. Watch for signs of low blood pressure. Get up slowly, and sit on the side of the bed to avoid dizziness. Check your blood pressure and pulse."
Acetaminophen (Tylenol): "Take this drug in recommended amounts for aches and general discomfort. Don't take aspirin because aspirin causes blood thinning and could upset your stomach."

(Continued on following page)

Box 4.4   METHOD DAILY TEACHING PLAN *(Continued)*

E (Environment): Assess patient for social supports to help him with self-care and transportation. Teach patient activity limitations while the patient is in the hospital, and find out activity prescription after discharge. Create an environment of trust and support so the patient can learn effectively.

T (Treatments): Demonstrate use of Accu-check, or have patient do procedure if ready. Use patient teaching aid booklet and video if available. Demonstrate insulin injection, or have patient self-administer if ready. Demonstrate care of equipment. Use patient teaching aid booklet and video if available. Describe skin care, wound care (if appropriate), and daily care of feet using teaching aids such as booklets or videos. Highlight information in patient teaching pamphlet: Use mild soap and lukewarm water; use lotions to keep skin soft; protect skin by using gloves while working and wearing sunscreen while outdoors; treat injuries immediately with soap, warm water, and dry sterile bandage; see physician or nurse practitioner if cuts do not heal or become infected (red, throbbing, warm, swelling, pus). Explain activity limitations, and have patient reiterate: "You will be out of bed to sit in a chair and walk with assistance today. Until your strength returns, you will need assistance to prevent falls."

H (Health Knowledge of Disease): "Hypoglycemia may be caused by taking in too much insulin, missing or delaying meals, exercising or working more than usual, or getting an infection or illness. It can develop rapidly, in 15 minutes to 1 hour. Symptoms include sweating, dizziness, shaking, hunger, or restlessness; numbness/tingling of the lips, tongue, hands, or feet; slurred speech, headache, or blurred vision. Carry candy or fruit juice with you, and drink it if you feel a hypoglycemic reaction coming. When the reaction is over, eat a serving of a slowly digested food such as cottage cheese, milk, or your scheduled meal or snack to prevent a second drop in blood sugar."

"Hyperglycemia can be caused by omitting insulin or taking less than the prescribed amount, eating more than the prescribed diet, or experiencing a great deal of stress. Illnesses with fever and infection may also cause hyperglycemia. Diabetic acidosis can result over hours or days. You had symptoms of hyperglycemia before coming into the hospital; they included excessive urination and thirst. You were tired, you lost weight, and you were dehydrated. Other signs and symptoms of hyperglycemia may include drowsiness, loss of appetite, blurred vision, abdominal pain, nausea, vomiting, and a fruity odor to your breath. To avoid hyperglycemia, follow your meal plan closely, test your blood glucose levels regularly, and report any consistently high levels. Call for an appointment with your physician or nurse practitioner when you have a fever or when a wound looks like it could be infected."

O (Outpatient/Inpatient Referrals): Sequential blood glucose monitoring: "The purpose of doing fingersticks with the glucometer before meals and at bedtime is to determine if the insulin and food you are taking is in the correct balance to control your blood glucose levels." Provide local and national resources.

D (Diet): 1800-calorie ADA diet, no added sugar. Attach sample menu and exchange lists. Include significant others in teaching meal planning and following exchange lists.

plan, assess him further to find out about his level of social support. Does he have family members or significant others to assist him at home and take him to follow-up appointments or diabetic education classes? Does he drive? While in the hospital, what special assistance did he need in his environment that he will still need at home? For example, does he need to be assisted with ambulation until his strength returns? He needs to be taught his activity restrictions while hospitalized. Therefore, the teaching plan could include the notations specified under Health Knowledge of Disease included in Box 4.4.

Treatments

The patient, someone in his family, or another person must learn to use the glucometer, draw up and give insulin, and keep records of the patient's blood glucose levels and the amount of insulin administered. These items on your teaching plan would look like Box 4.4, listed under Treatments. Give the patient written instructions for how to use the glucometer and how to administer insulin. As you demonstrate how to check blood glucose levels and give an insulin injection, provide simple instructions for each step. Then ask the patient to give you a return demonstration, in which he tries to use the glucometer and give himself an insulin injection. Reassure and help him; he will be anxious at first.

Also, explain and demonstrate what the patient needs to do to care for his skin and feet. Again, have him give you a return demonstration. If the patient's nurse has already taught him these skills, check his understanding by asking him questions or watching him demonstrate them.

Health Knowledge of Disease

The patient needs to know the signs and symptoms of his disease and when it is time to call the physician or nurse practitioner. In this case, it is most important for the patient to know about hypoglycemia and hyperglycemia and what to do about these conditions when they occur. Review the signs and symptoms of hypoglycemia and hyperglycemia with the patient, and explain the circumstances most likely to precipitate symptoms. Again, consult Box 4.4, Health Knowledge of Disease, for an example of what your teaching plan might say.

Inpatient and Outpatient Referrals

Be prepared to explain any test or procedure in a sentence or two using nonmedical terminology. This particular patient is not scheduled for any blood tests in addition to his blood glucose levels. But be prepared to explain when, where, how, and why sequential blood glucose tests are needed as applicable to the patient situation, as described in Box 4.4.

There is no way to predict what other tests will be ordered, and you are not expected to memorize every test. The more common tests will become very familiar as your experiences and knowledge increase. An overview of some common tests with normal values was described in Chapter 2. There will always be references available to look up laboratory tests and procedures on your unit. You can also call the laboratory or department in which the test is to be done and request information materials for the test or procedure.

It is helpful to give patients information on local and national resources concerning their health problems. The Internet is an excellent resource for locating addresses or phone numbers of agencies so that patients and their significant others have a place to start looking for more information if they are interested. For example, national diabetes resources include:

▶ American Diabetes Association National Service Center, 1660 Duke Street, Alexandria VA 22314; 1-800-DIABETES (1-800-342-2383); http://www.diabetes.org/default.htm
▶ Diabetes resources on the Internet: http://vigora.com/resources/
▶ National Diabetes Information Clearinghouse, 1 Information Way, Bethesda MD 20892-3570; http://www.niddk.nih.gov/health/diabetes/ndic.htm

Once you know what the national organizations are, look in the phone book to determine whether there is a local branch of the organization. If so, provide the patient or significant other with the appropriate phone numbers.

At this point in your planning process, you have no specific data about the patient's discharge. The physician or nurse practitioner will provide instructions for scheduling follow-up appointments and arranging for a home health care agency, if necessary.

Diet

This patient has been prescribed an 1800-calorie ADA diet with no added sugar. You will need to teach him how to use a food exchange list. Fruits, breads, meats, fats, and milk products are grouped in lists. Exchange lists and sample menus may be obtained from the dietary department in the health-care agency. You can also obtain online information from the American Dietetic Association. The American Dietetic Association is the professional organization of dietitians, the same as the ANA is for nurses. The most current recommendations for nutrition are available from this organization.

Plan to sit down with the patient to discuss the diet and the food lists. Ask him to plan his meals according to what he likes to eat, using the exchange lists. Plan to have significant others also hear your instructions, especially the person who usually prepares the patient's meals.

The preceding discussion of the teaching plan includes details of teaching content and rationales. Your mini–teaching plan should be no more than about one page long. It should provide an outline of what you will need to teach. Attach all relevant teaching materials you will be using.

There is no need to rewrite and duplicate information found in the teaching materials and standardized care plans. The plan should contain the information listed in Box 4.4.

In summary, the METHOD daily teaching plan is a focused, individualized plan based on data from the concept care maps and general standardized teaching plans. You are expected to attach relevant teaching materials to the plan.

Developing Teaching Skills

To be an effective teacher, you must know not only what to teach but also how to teach it. You must assess the patient and significant others for learning readiness before trying to teach anything. For example, if the patient is highly anxious or in considerable pain, or if he is tired or hungry, you may try to teach him something; however, chances are that he will retain little of the information you provide, and he may become even more anxious.

To teach effectively, you will need to use basic principles of teaching and learning in adults and children, and you will need to use key adult learning principles, teaching strategies, and evaluation methods (Box 4.5). For further discussion of basic principles of learning and teaching strategies, refer to Chapter 9 in *Communication:*

Box 4.5   ADULT LEARNING PRINCIPLES

Use these principles when teaching adult patients:

- Build on previous experiences.
- Focus on immediate concerns first.
- Adapt teaching to the patient's lifestyle.
- Make the patient an active participant.
- Determine learning readiness.
- Be realistic, and stick to the basics.
- Take advantage of the teachable moment by incorporating teaching into your ongoing patient care.
- Reinforce all learning.
- Solicit feedback.

Knowledge-Based Teaching Strategies

Your teaching methods must coincide with the type of knowledge you are trying to convey. Use these techniques:

- *Cognitive knowledge (facts):* Give explanations and descriptions; use books, pamphlets, films, programmed instruction, and computer programs.
- *Affective and cognitive knowledge (feelings and beliefs):* Use one-to-one discussions, group discussions, role-

playing, and discovery to guide the patient in problem-solving situations to help him express feelings and use cognitive knowledge to solve problems.
▶ *Psychomotor knowledge (skills):* Use demonstrations accompanied by explanations.

Evaluation of Teaching: Did the Patient Learn?

To assess your patient's learning, use these techniques:

▶ *Cognitive knowledge:* Ask oral or written questions; ask the patient to keep a diary or records of self-monitoring.
▶ *Affective knowledge:* Infer the patient's level of learning from how he responds to you, how he speaks about his illness and his treatments, and how he verbally expresses his feelings and values.
▶ *Psychomotor knowledge:* Ask the patient for a return demonstration.

The Key to the Therapeutic Relationship by Schuster. Therapeutic communication is the foundation of the nurse-patient relationship. You must know how to use therapeutic communication throughout the process of teaching.

Teaching plans focus on data from the concept care map and on general patient teaching information prioritized to address the most important problems first. Keep in mind that anxiety blocks communication and learning and that even a calm patient can only absorb so much information at one time. When possible, ask the patient where he would like to start, and then be flexible. Bring your detailed, standardized care plans with you, and refer to them if the patient asks questions you are not prepared to answer. Students are not expected to know every aspect of teaching about every health problem. As needed, refer questions to your clinical faculty, cover nurse, or to the appropriate health-care personnel, such as the diabetes educator or dietitian in this example.

CHAPTER 4 SUMMARY

The purpose of this chapter was to guide you in the development of step 4 of the concept care map development. Step 4 involves prioritizing and then developing goals, outcomes, and nursing interventions for each diagnosis. Nursing interventions are developed to support patients physically and emotionally and to provide the services that patients cannot provide for themselves. Emotional support through therapeutic communication is as important as the physical care provided to patients.

Step 4 is based on thinking critically and synthesizing information from standardized care plans and the data available on the concept care map. Step 4 also involves developing a teaching plan for the patient and significant others. The components of the teaching plan for the day of care can be remembered using the acronym METHOD. These letters stand for the key elements of a teaching plan: medications, environment, treatments, health knowledge, outpatient/inpatient referrals, and diet.

Carry your concept care map, goals, objectives, outcomes, interventions, and teaching plan in your pocket on the clinical unit. Also, bring the standardized care plans, clinical pathways (if available), medication cards or printouts, and relevant patient education teaching materials as needed. In addition, bring the patient profile database with the falls-risk assessment and pressure ulcer risk scale assessment. What you need to bring to the clinical site is listed in Box 4.6.

Box 4.6	CHECKLIST: WHAT TO BRING TO THE CLINICAL AGENCY

1. Patient profile database
2. Concept map based on patient profile database (steps 1–3)
3. Plan of goals/outcomes/interventions (step 4)
4. Pressure ulcer risk assessment scale
5. Falls-risk assessment scale
6. METHOD teaching plan
7. Patient education materials
8. Standardized care plans
9. Clinical pathways, if available
10. Printouts or medication cards for all drugs

LEARNING ACTIVITIES

To do these exercises, you will need access to books on medical-surgical nursing, nutrition, medications, diagnostic tests and procedures, and standardized care plans. One approach is to form a group ahead of time and have each person bring a specific reference to class instead of having each student carry all of the references.

1. Work in groups of three to four students to develop step 4 goals, outcomes, and interventions for patient scenarios 2 and 3, which appear in the end-of-chapter exercises for Chapter 3. Split up the diagnoses among the groups. Each group should write its goals, outcomes, and interventions on the board for critique by the entire class.

2. A representative of each group should state rationales for the interventions for the assigned diagnosis.

3. Develop METHOD teaching plans for patient scenarios 2 and 3. Split up the components of the teaching plan (medications, environment, treatments, health knowledge, outpatient/inpatient referrals, and diet) among the group. Write the teaching components on the board so the entire class can critique the content of the teaching plan.

4. A representative of each group should state the teaching methods that would be used to teach the information.

5. Using the diabetic patient in this chapter as an example, explain what you would say and do to assess his anxiety, show empathy, and use therapeutic touch and therapeutic humor.

6. Using the exchange list from this chapter, practice making a sample meal for the diabetic patient on an 1800-calorie ADA diet with no added sugar. What could he eat for breakfast, lunch, supper, and snack? Which foods should he avoid?

REFERENCES

1. Nursing's Social Policy Statement, ed 2. American Nurses Association, nursesbooks.org, Washington, D.C., 2003.
2. Schuster, PM: Communication: The Key to the Therapeutic Relationship. FA Davis, Philadelphia, 2000.
3. Ibid.
4. Huey, R, et al: Discharge planning: Good planning means fewer hospitalizations for the chronically ill. Nursing 81:11-20, 1981. (This is a classic seminal article.)

NURSING IMPLEMENTATION:
Using Concept Care Maps as Nursing Care Plans at the Health-Care Agency

OBJECTIVES

1. Describe clinical organizational strategies necessary for successful clinical performance.

2. Identify American Nurses Association (ANA) Standards of Clinical Nursing Practice related to implementation and evaluation of nursing care plans in the health-care agency.

3. Describe how to update and modify a concept care map upon arrival at the clinical agency.

4. Relate how to use a concept care map during interactions with patients.

5. Describe the evaluation of patient responses to nursing interventions done during step 5 of the concept care map.

6. Describe how the concept care map can be used to facilitate communication between the student nurse, the clinical faculty, and the patient's staff nurse.

7. Use the concept care map to explain the relationship between medications and relevant clinical data before giving drugs.

8. Describe the development of concept care maps for use in outpatient settings.

The concept care map is used as an organizational tool for clinical data. A focus of this chapter is on organizational strategies to prioritize what must be done during a clinical day to implement the plan of care. This chapter also describes implementation and evaluation of nursing care using the concept care map.

Standard 6 of the ANA Standards of Clinical Nursing Practice mandates that nurses take responsibility for the implementation of interventions identified in the nursing care plan.[1] In the clinical setting, the concept care map becomes a dynamic working clinical patient care tool to assist you with organizing the data for the ongoing care of your patients.

Standard 7 of the ANA Standards of Clinical Nursing Practice requires that nurses and patients take responsibility for evaluating patients' progress toward attaining their outcomes and goals.[2] This is accomplished by identifying patient responses to interventions, which is step 5 of the concept care map. You must discipline yourself to focus carefully on and evaluate patient responses to each intervention, and you must record these responses on the concept care map. In addition, you must also determine the patient's viewpoint regarding his or her progress toward the outcome objectives.

Standard 8 of the ANA Standards of Clinical Nursing Practice mandates that the nurse revise the nursing plan of care, reassess, reorder priorities, and establish new goals, outcomes, and interventions as needed to maximize the patient's health capabilities.[3] Therefore, you must be able to update the concept care map to account for dynamic changes that regularly occur in clinical settings. You will face many challenges throughout a clinical day. Nothing ever goes exactly as planned!

Arrival in the Inpatient Unit: Getting Organized

Getting organized is crucial for successful clinical performance. When you arrive at the clinical unit, you must obtain the latest data for medications, intravenous (IV) fluids, and treatments, along with a patient status report. Write updates directly on your concept care map "sloppy

| Box 5.1 | WHAT TO DO WHEN YOU ARRIVE AT THE UNIT |

1. Check the patient's medication record.
2. Check the patient's IV administration record.
3. Check the patient's treatments.
4. Check the patient's laboratory data.
5. Obtain a patient report from the preceding shift.

copy." Put new data on the "sloppy copy" under the appropriate diagnoses. Do not use a separate sheet of paper for the updates because a separate sheet of paper could easily get lost. Use a red pen so you and your clinical faculty can quickly see your revisions. A prioritized list of all the activities you must complete to update your plan of care is shown in Box 5.1.

Check Medication Records

Check for changes in the patient's medications by reviewing medication records for routine and as-needed (prn) drugs. Update your concept care map by adding, deleting, or revising drugs. Write the times at which medications should be administered on the front of the map in red ink. Highlight medications so you can find them easily on the concept care map. Write on the concept care map what time the patient last received a prn pain medication as well as the name of the drug. If you are not familiar with any of the drugs the patient is receiving, before giving the medications look them up in a drug reference book, or call the pharmacy to obtain information.

Check IV Administration Records

Check for changes in the patient's IV records. Record the current fluid being administered and rate of administration on the concept care map diagram in the appropriate nursing diagnosis box. Highlight the IV fluid and rate of administration. Also note and highlight admixtures and length of infusion time.

Check Treatments

Check for updates in the patient's treatments, and write these on the concept care map in the appropriate nursing diagnosis box. If the information does not fit in any of the diagnostic boxes that appear on the map, make a new diagnosis box. If you are not sure where the new information goes, place it in the box labeled "I don't know how this fits with the problems," and check with your clinical faculty.

Check Laboratory Data

Check the records for laboratory tests and diagnostic procedures that were ordered from the time you left the unit. Find out which laboratory tests and procedures were completed and which reports are pending. For completed laboratory tests and procedures, find the reports, and write the results on your concept care map in the appropriate diagnostic categories. For pending laboratory results, write the name of the test, and place a blank next to it so you will know to fill in the result when it becomes available. Typically, the daily morning blood work is drawn between 5 and 6 a.m., and laboratory reports come back to the units early. You must have the latest information on laboratory data before administering many of the patient's drugs. For example, if you need to give Lanoxin (digoxin) and Lasix (furosemide), you will first need to know the most recent potassium value.

It is also crucial to analyze blood samples that are related to medications, because side effects of medications are often detected through analysis of blood samples. In this example, Lasix causes potassium to be lost in the urine. Hypokalemia may result in digitalis toxicity.

Obtain Information From the Previous Shift

There is always an end-of-shift summary report for each patient. It is crucial that you obtain a report of the patient's recent health status. Change-of-shift reports may take many different forms, including:

- A verbal report, with all oncoming nursing staff members taking notes on all patients
- Tape-recorded reports
- Written reports
- Verbal one-on-one reports between the nurse who is leaving and the nurse who is starting to deliver care to a particular group of patients

Write the information you obtain from the change-of-shift report in the appropriate nursing diagnosis boxes on your map. If necessary, make a new box if the data suggest a new nursing diagnosis. If you do not know where new information belongs on your map, put it in the box labeled "I don't know how this fits with the problems.," and check with your clinical faculty.

In short, as soon as you get to the healthcare agency, start collecting data to update your concept care map sloppy copy. Obtain data from medication records, IV records, treatments, laboratory data, and staff nurses. Look at the laboratory data that were collected while you were gone, and note any laboratory data that are pending. Medications are usually the priority; many (such as insulin and Lasix) must be given on time. It is also important to give pain medications on time. Always check medications first, because you may need to give a medication before doing anything else.

The nurses at the end of their shifts will be busy finishing their documentation and preparing their reports for the oncoming shift. This is not a good time to ask them questions. The outgoing nurses will give you and the oncoming nurses shift report as scheduled when they have completed their work. After the shift report, you may ask them additional questions before they leave.

Clinical Preconference

For many students, a clinical preconference is held early in the clinical day, after the change-of-shift report. The purpose of the preconference is for clinical faculty to meet with students to review the accuracy of the concept care map. By looking at your concept care map, your clinical faculty will be able to see very quickly if you have collected, correctly analyzed, categorized, and prioritized data. Goals, outcomes, and interventions are reviewed quickly. Succinct lists on a concept care map facilitate a rapid evaluation of the plan of care.

You must be prepared to address questions concerning your plan of care. This includes assessment data, nursing and medical diagnoses, goals, outcomes, interventions, and rationales. Your faculty may prefer that you write out rationales for all interventions. After the preconference, keep the concept care map in your pocket to guide you throughout the day.

Updating Assessments, Reporting Findings, Giving Medications

After determining your initial priorities and completing your preconference, you will most likely need to accomplish several more specific tasks (Box 5.2). These tasks include patient assessment, reporting the findings of your assessment, and preparing to give medications.

Patient Assessment and Evaluation

If the patient is sleeping, wake him to do your first assessment of the clinical day. If you are like many beginning students, you may not want to disturb the patient's sleep. It is critical, however, that you have the assessment data you need to make sound clinical judgments. In fact, it is pos-

sible that the patient is not sleeping but is comatose, and you would not know that unless you attempted to awaken him. A diabetic patient could be unconscious from hypoglycemia. It is a professional standard of care that assessments are done on each patient early at the start of each shift. Write your findings in the evaluation column of your care plan, shown in Figure 5.1. The recorded notes of patient responses fall under step 5 of the concept care map. These notes will be the basis of documentation that will be explained in Chapter 7. Start your assessments by performing the key assessments first. If your patient needs to go for a test, or if your instructor, his doctor, or nurse comes in to see the patient, you will be able to report your findings. All health-care providers will want to know the key assessments, so always do the key assessments first, because they are the most important. The key assessments for the newly diagnosed patient with diabetes are signs and symptoms of hypoglycemia and hyperglycemia, blood glucose value, food intake and vital signs. The key assessments that you must do first are going to be different for each patient. It is important to note that the patient response is to be recorded, not that you did the intervention. The patient response to your intervention is based on your evaluation and continual assessment of the patient. The recorded notes of patient responses comprise step 5 of the concept care map.

Reporting Assessment Data

Once you have done your assessment and evaluation and have taken notes, find your patient's assigned staff nurse, introduce yourself if necessary, and report your assessment findings. If you happen to see your clinical faculty before you see the patient's nurse, report your findings to the clinical faculty. Assessment and patient evaluation involves critical information that both your faculty and patient's assigned staff nurse want to know as soon as possible during the first hour of the shift.

Once the patient's immediate needs are met, review with the patient's assigned staff nurse what you will and will not be doing for patient care. You may need to say, "I don't know how to do the dressing change yet." or "I haven't learned to use the glucometer." The staff nurse is respon-

Box 5.2 WHAT TO DO AFTER UPDATING THE CARE PLAN

1. Perform patient assessment.
2. Report assessment data to patient's assigned staff nurse.
3. Report assessment data to clinical faculty.
4. Locate medications.
5. Meet faculty in medication area to prepare for drug administration (if applicable).

Problem #_____1_____ : Imbalanced Nutrition: Less than body requirements
General Goal: To improve the patient's nutritional status

Predicted Behavioral Outcome Objective (s): The patient will...maintain his blood glucose between 80 and 120 mg/dl by eating his 1800-calorie ADA diet and administering insulin injections as scheduled...on the day of care.

Nursing Interventions	Patient Responses to Interventions
1. Assess abdomen: bowel sounds, tenderness, distention, BMs	1. BS all quads, nontender, nondistended, no BM
2. Assess blood glucose with glucometer at 0800 and 1100	2. 60 at 7:30, 100 at 11:30
3. Assess S/S of hypoglycemia and hyperglycemia	3. 7:45, clammy/sweaty, dizzy, hungry
4. Monitor appetite–1800 cal ADA, no sugar added	4. Ate 90% breakfast, 50% lunch
5. Measure fluid intake and output	5. I=400, 350, 200 0=250, 225, 300
6. Administer insulin on time	6. 8:00 insulin held, Dr. notified, continue glucometer measurements and call for further orders after each BS
7. Check for additional blood work	7. K=3.8
8. Monitor patient for orthostatic hypotension and weakness	8. Steady while standing and walking BP 124/60 standing
9. Ambulate carefully to avoid falls	9. Able to walk without assistance to BR

Evaluation: Summarize patient progress toward outcome objectives: Need to continue to carefully monitor for hypoglycemia and hyperglycemia because diet, insulin, and blood sugar still not coordinated, is stronger and is cautious with movement.

Problem #_____2_____ : Anxiety
General Goal: Decrease anxiety

Predicted Behavioral Outcome Objective (s): The patient will...verbalize concerns about his disease and the changes that must be made in his lifestyle...on the day of care.

Nursing Interventions	Patient Responses to Interventions
1. Assess current level of anxiety	1. Appeared anxious during hypoglycemic episode
2. Use empathy	2. Verbalized concerns about disease
3. Use therapeutic touch	3. Accepted touch, eased anxiety
4. Use therapeutic humor	4. Responded by smiling, eased anxiety

Evaluation: Summarize patient progress toward outcome objectives: Patient stated he was concerned about learning how to give his own injections and how to prepare meals. Therapeutic communication techniques effective in gaining cooperation and mutual goal setting, and helped to control anxiety by verbalization of concerns.

Problem #_____3_____ : Deficient knowledge
General Goal: Increase knowledge

Predicted Behavioral Outcome Objective (s): The patient will...decide in collaboration with the nurse what aspects of diabetic teaching protocol he would like to focus on during... the day of care.

Nursing Interventions	Patient Responses to Interventions
1. Assess current level of knowledge and establish what the patient most wants to learn about during the day of care	1. Wants to know about hypoglycemia, glucometer monitoring, and insulin injections
2. Assess resources available for teaching, such as diabetic educator, dietitian, programs, or movies	2. Diabetes educator visited and will start classes at outpatient clinic when discharged
3. See teaching plan for: –what diabetes is and how it affects health (signs and symptoms) –Medications –Diet –Skin care –Exercise/activity	3. Focused on signs and symptoms, use of glucometer, drawing up insulin, see teaching plan for evaluation of teaching

Evaluation: Summarize patient progress toward outcome objectives: Needs continued practice to use glucometer. Did not need insulin this shift so could not practice self-administration. Did correctly draw up the medication. Can state the signs of hypoglycemia and hyperglycemia. Review of menus not done due to lack of time.

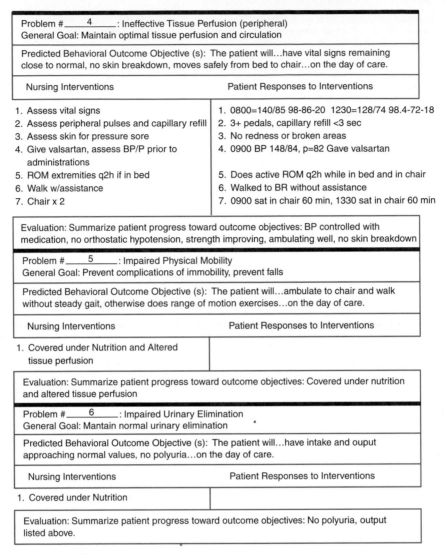

Problem #____4____: Ineffective Tissue Perfusion (peripheral)
General Goal: Maintain optimal tissue perfusion and circulation

Predicted Behavioral Outcome Objective (s): The patient will...have vital signs remaining close to normal, no skin breakdown, moves safely from bed to chair...on the day of care.

Nursing Interventions	Patient Responses to Interventions
1. Assess vital signs	1. 0800=140/85 98-86-20 1230=128/74 98.4-72-18
2. Assess peripheral pulses and capillary refill	2. 3+ pedals, capillary refill <3 sec
3. Assess skin for pressure sore	3. No redness or broken areas
4. Give valsartan, assess BP/P prior to administrations	4. 0900 BP 148/84, p=82 Gave valsartan
5. ROM extremities q2h if in bed	5. Does active ROM q2h while in bed and in chair
6. Walk w/assistance	6. Walked to BR without assistance
7. Chair x 2	7. 0900 sat in chair 60 min, 1330 sat in chair 60 min

Evaluation: Summarize patient progress toward outcome objectives: BP controlled with medication, no orthostatic hypotension, strength improving, ambulating well, no skin breakdown

Problem #____5____: Impaired Physical Mobility
General Goal: Prevent complications of immobility, prevent falls

Predicted Behavioral Outcome Objective (s): The patient will...ambulate to chair and walk without steady gait, otherwise does range of motion exercises...on the day of care.

Nursing Interventions	Patient Responses to Interventions
1. Covered under Nutrition and Altered tissue perfusion	

Evaluation: Summarize patient progress toward outcome objectives: Covered under nutrition and altered tissue perfusion

Problem #____6____: Impaired Urinary Elimination
General Goal: Maintain normal urinary elimination

Predicted Behavioral Outcome Objective (s): The patient will...have intake and ouput approaching normal values, no polyuria...on the day of care.

Nursing Interventions	Patient Responses to Interventions
1. Covered under Nutrition	

Evaluation: Summarize patient progress toward outcome objectives: No polyuria, output listed above.

● Figure 5.1   Steps 4 and 5 of the concept care map.

sible for doing what you have not yet learned to do, so you must be very clear about what you can do and what the nurse will need to do. She may review the daily plan of care with you, emphasizing from her viewpoint the important aspects of care that must be done.

Communication must flow openly between you, the faculty, and the patient's staff nurse.

Any time you find abnormalities in any of your patient's assessment data (be sure to report abnormal key assessment data first), interrupt the staff nurse or your clinical faculty to report the abnormality. The key words here are *interrupt* and *abnormalities*. Abnormalities include anything not within normal parameters. For

example, a blood pressure of 150/92 is not within normal parameters. Many students hesitate to interrupt when the faculty or staff nurse looks busy. Get the attention of one or the other no matter how busy they might appear. Abnormal assessment data mean the patient could be in trouble, and the staff nurse and clinical faculty have the knowledge to make a clinical judgment about what is an imminent danger and what can wait until later. Each of these nurses will want to personally assess and evaluate the patient's responses to validate your findings.

Even if you find and interrupt your clinical faculty and she tells you that she cannot come to the patient's bedside immediately, she will tell you to find the patient's assigned staff nurse or the charge nurse. She will check on you and your patient as soon as possible. If the staff nurse and clinical faculty are both too busy, they will refer you to yet another nurse.

Finding Medications

After the assessment and report phase, the next step is to find all your medications for the shift. You already checked the medication administration record and made updates. Now you actually have to find the drugs. Check to make sure all the pills, injections, liquids, eyedrops, inhalants, IV medications, and other required items are on the unit. Medications may be in a medication cart, a refrigerator, or at the bedside. Some may come from a computerized dispenser. Carefully check all currently available drugs. For a drug that is not normally kept on the unit, you may need to follow hospital policy to obtain it. To do so, you may need to call the pharmacy, fax an order, or go to the pharmacy to pick up the drug. Once you have found all your patient's medications, meet your clinical faculty in the medication area early in the shift to discuss administration.

The concept care map is particularly useful as you and your clinical faculty analyze relationships between the patient's laboratory data, physical assessment data, and medications. For example, the discussion of the relationship between insulin, blood glucose level, and appetite is facilitated because all these items are in the same diagnostic box. Likewise, a discussion of the need to assess the patient's blood pressure before giving the antihypertensive drug valsartan (Diovan) is apparent because they are in the same box. When you see drugs, laboratory work, and physical assessment data in proximity, the relationships are defined in your mind. You will soon realize that you must know the blood glucose level to decide whether to give the patient his insulin. If his blood glucose level is too low, you could harm the patient by giving the drug.

Using the Concept Care Map to Facilitate Communication

The concept care map is a bridge that facilitates communication between you and faculty. As clinical faculty make bedside rounds, the concept care map allows you to easily discuss the patient's progress toward or away from goals and outcomes. As a result of your discussion, you can make notes and revisions on the concept care map or nursing intervention lists.

Bedside Communication

Bedside rounds occur periodically throughout the day. Assessment data can be validated by your faculty or staff nurse or corrected if inaccurate, and concept care maps can be updated as a result of rounds. Faculty comments should appear on your map in a distinct color, such as purple or green, so that these comments are easily visible. Faculty may make written notations instructing you to continue to assess certain aspects of care, to try specific interventions, or to illustrate the finer aspects of the interrelationships of care. Because concept care maps show a comprehensive patient picture, they facilitate a thorough discussion between you and your faculty.

For example, the clinical faculty might walk into the room and say: "Let's see your diagram on the sloppy copy, patient objectives, and intervention lists." The faculty may then proceed to ask questions such as: "How is he eating? What's his last blood glucose? Any signs of hypoglycemia? How much is he urinating? How's his blood pressure and pulse? What have you covered so far in your teaching?" These questions can be addressed by reviewing the updated concept care map.

Reporting Off the Unit

You are responsible to report to the patient's assigned staff nurse before going on breaks and before going home. Never leave a unit without giving a report to the patient's assigned staff nurse. Focus the report on the key areas of assessment that are most crucial to the care of the patient, located centrally on the diagram under the reason for admission to the healthcare facility. If anything is abnormal, be sure to tell the staff nurse. Get out your concept care map, and use it to remind yourself what you need to say. For example, as you go to lunch at 11:40 a.m., tell the staff nurse, "He hasn't had any more signs of hypoglycemia and the 11:30 a.m. fingerstick was 100. He did it himself, but he still can't remember the exact procedure without help. The doctor wants to be notified about the glucose. The patient is eating in bed right now. Everything else is fine."

Implementation for the Diabetic Patient

The diabetic patient who appeared in earlier chapters will help to illustrate the process of

organizing, implementing, and evaluating patient care. Start by reviewing the concept care map in Figure 5.2. It has been updated from a review of patient records and the shift report. On the concept care map diagram, medications are highlighted to make them more prominent.

Assessment

First, you must do a head-to-toe physical assessment of the patient. Focus initially on assessing what you have determined to be essential key assessments, which are written in the center box

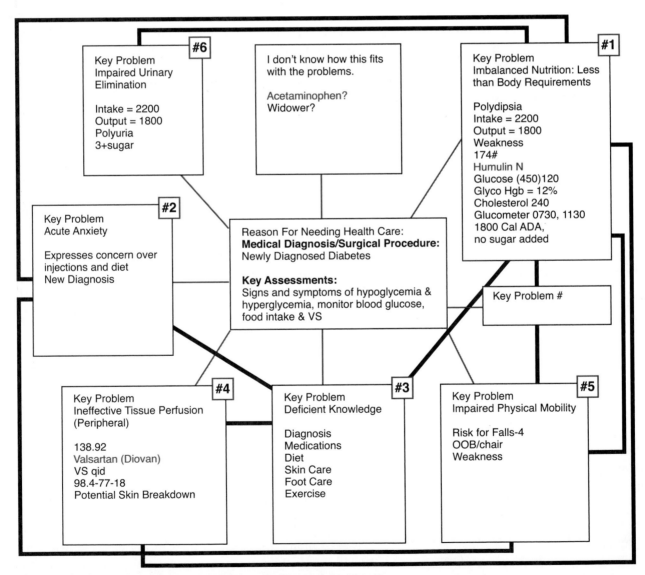

● Figure 5.2   Highlight your patient's medications on the diagram.

on your concept care map under the patient's reason for needing health care. A head-to-toe assessment is the most important way to obtain baseline data at the start of the shift. You must be thorough. For example, if you check a patient's lungs, check all lung fields. Student nurses sometimes hesitate to "disturb" a patient to do a complete assessment. The patient may be in pain, he may be immobilized for any number of reasons, or he may simply be asleep. If necessary, get an assistant to hold the patient up while you assess all lung fields and perform the rest of your assessment. Physical assessments are done at least once a shift, more often if the patient's acuity level makes them necessary.

For your diabetic patient, ask him about signs and symptoms of hypoglycemia and hyperglycemia, obtain results of his blood glucose test, and ask about food intake. As you greet the patient with a handshake, start with a general question, such as, "How are you doing this morning?" Listen carefully to see if the patient says anything that could suggest a problem.

Consider this scenario: He keeps hold of your hand and says that he feels sweaty and light-headed this morning. He is responding to your touch by holding onto you. You ask if he is hungry. He says yes. You ask if he is feeling numb anywhere. He says no. You say, "I'll check your blood sugar and see what it is." You then check his blood glucose level using the glucometer and find it to be 60. You also find that his blood pressure is 140/85, his pulse is 86, and his respirations are 20. Quickly write the blood glucose level and vital signs on the care plan so you do not forget them.

From these data, you conclude that the patient is hypoglycemic but stable. You ask if he can eat his breakfast, and he says yes. You get the tray, open some orange juice for him, and watch while he drinks it. If the tray is not yet available, you can get him orange juice and crackers. Then you immediately report what happened to the patient's staff nurse and your clinical faculty. Recount the patient's report of symptoms, the blood glucose level, the vital signs, and what you did about the patient's problem.

Suppose you do not know how to use the glucometer. In that case, take the patient's blood pressure, pulse, and respirations, and conclude from his report that he is probably hypoglycemic but has stable vital signs. Immediately ask your faculty or the patient's staff nurse to check his blood glucose level. Tell the staff nurse you have not yet learned to use the glucometer, and ask her to do it. You will have the staff nurse's immediate, undivided attention if you tell her the patient is having a hypoglycemic reaction. This problem needs immediate attention in order to intervene before it gets any worse.

Establish Mutual Goals

After performing your assessment, negotiate with the patient to establish mutual goals, expected outcomes, and a schedule of activities. Use the list of goals, outcomes, and interventions that you constructed and, in very simple terms, review with the patient what needs to be done. Discuss each of the problems, and listen carefully to what the patient believes should be the goals and outcomes of care for the day.

For example, you know that the patient needs to do morning care, to get up safely into a chair, to learn about self-care and diabetes, and especially to learn what to do about hypoglycemic reactions. As you review with the patient, use empathy and humor to establish a therapeutic relationship. By using therapeutic communication techniques, you will be better able to find out what the patient is thinking. For instance, you may discover that he is especially concerned about fluctuations in his blood glucose levels and regulation of insulin with his meals. Of course, you will have things that you consider to be important. You will want to discuss his weakness and his risk of falling. Tell him to be cautious when getting up, and explain that you want to be present when he does get up so you can check his blood pressure. List the major items the patient needs to learn for self-care, and let the patient select which aspects of teaching he wants to start with. This portion of the day is about establishing agreements and goals. A successful outcome of your conversation with him thus far would be for him to say that he will not get out of bed without calling you and that he wants to learn how to check his blood glucose after morning care. The goals, outcomes, and interventions you established will guide your discussions with the patient in the morning and throughout the day.

Implementing and Evaluating Care

Make sure you do everything you said you were going to do on your plan of care. Some students prefer to check off each item in the list of interventions as they do them so they do not forget to do anything. Your clinical faculty and the patient's staff nurse will be expecting you to either carry out each nursing intervention you listed in step 4 or report that it could not be completed in a timely manner. For example, suppose you write that the patient is to do range-of-motion exercises every 2 hours. You are responsible for checking every two hours and for reminding the patient to do these exercises if he forgets. Failure to carry out all established interventions as planned and in a timely manner is negligent, is a breach of the standards of care, and considered malpractice. Therefore, make sure you keep your faculty informed, no matter how busy they may appear.

As you perform interventions, evaluate the patient's responses to assess his progress toward expected outcomes throughout the day. Record these responses in a different colored ink in the column across from your intervention list (see Fig. 5.1).

Step 5 includes writing an evaluation summary of the patient's progress toward the outcome objectives. This summary includes your clinical judgments. Carefully consider the effectiveness of your interventions in bringing about the expected patient outcomes. If your interventions are not working and the patient is not progressing as anticipated, your clinical faculty and the patient's assigned staff nurse are there to help you consider other interventions and to make revisions in the concept care map.

Evaluate the patient's verbal and nonverbal behaviors regarding each item on the intervention list throughout the day. Also consider physical assessment data. Take notes as you go along. You will probably not be doing the interventions in the order you have written them on the intervention "to do" lists, but that is fine. Because interventions are not done in order, you should check off each item as you do it to keep track of what has been done.

Evaluation of the Teaching Plan

Your teaching plan must be evaluated like your basic care plan (see Box 4.4 in Chapter 4 to review the teaching plan). Focus on teaching methods, responses of the patient or significant others to teaching, and knowledge gained by the patient (Box 5.3). Also note what should be taught and what should be reinforced by the patient's next nurse to ensure continuity of care.

Other Outcomes to Review

Evaluate the patient's outcomes against standardized care plans and clinical paths. As you evaluate, you learn to predict expected patient responses, and you can judge how removed your patient is from the expectations for the "typical" patient. Nurses use standardized plans and clinical paths to double-check that everything that was supposed to be done was done. In addition, falls and skin assessments with expected outcomes must be evaluated.

Inpatient Versus Outpatient Settings

An obvious difference between inpatient and outpatient units is the acuity level of the patients. Although patients are typically healthier in outpatient settings, you will still need to perform careful assessments, make nursing diagnoses, establish outcomes, perform interventions, and evaluate patient responses. It is not possible to complete an individualized care plan ahead of time for an outpatient. Standardized plans of care and clinical pathways are used as guides for outpatient care. Preparation for an outpatient visit involves reviewing the typical procedures and plans of care that are used in the outpatient setting.

For example, in an endoscopy department, you would review the department's endoscopy procedure flow sheets, preprocedure and postprocedure orders, standardized discharge instructions, and conscious sedation flow sheets. You could use a medical-surgical textbook to review general symptoms and typical diseases

Box 5.3   EVALUATION OF TEACHING PLAN

Evaluation of Patient Education
Teaching techniques:
Evaluation: Used discussion, question and
answers, and demonstrations
M (Medications)
Evaluation: Discussed each medication.
Patient knew the purpose of each drug.
Was checking his own blood pressure
each week at home using cuff he bought
at the drugstore. Needs to review side
effects and precautions of insulin and
valsartan. Received printed drug information.
E (Environment)
Evaluation: Patient lives next door to his
son, who checks on him daily and will
help with meals, medication administration, getting to appointments, and so
on. Verbalizes activity restrictions in
the hospital.
T (Treatments)
Evaluation: Glucometer demonstrated,
and patient did his own fingerstick.

Received printed instructions for oper-
ating machine. Insulin not given, but
patient drew up practice dose without
assistance.
H (Health Knowledge of Disease)
Evaluation: Verbalizes signs and symptoms of hypoglycemia and hyperglycemia. States what to do to avoid
hypoglycemia and hyperglycemia.
Relates symptoms experienced in morning to signs and symptoms of hypoglycemia.
O (Outpatient/Inpatient Referrals)
Evaluation: States purpose of doing fingersticks and sequential monitoring.
Received information for national and
regional resources.
D (Diet)
Evaluation: Patient was tired and needed
a rest, thus unable to finish diet teaching. Information given to nurse who will
be doing evening care. Planning to
teach diet with son in attendance.

diagnosed using endoscopy procedures. You also must be aware of possible complications during and after the procedure and carefully monitor patients throughout their time in the department. After reviewing these materials, it would be possible for you to make predictions about possible key nursing diagnoses and develop a concept care map that might look like Figure 5.3.

Once you and the patient arrive on the endoscopy outpatient unit, you must gather assessment data. For example, Figure 5.4 illustrates information gathered from a 47-year-old woman before she had an endoscopy procedure in the outpatient department.

During the procedure, the patient's blood pressure, pulses, respirations, pulse oximetry, and level of consciousness will be carefully monitored. She will receive drugs for sedation and pain. After the procedure, the nurse will perform

a head-to-toe assessment, with special consideration for the gastrointestinal system and elimination. The nurse will be sure the following attained these outcomes before discharge:

- Stable vital signs
- Patent airway
- Intact gag reflex
- Minimal nausea, vomiting, and dizziness
- Oral fluids tolerated
- Able to ambulate
- Able to void
- Comfortable pain level
- Understands home-going instructions

The pace of care in outpatient settings is very rapid. The nurses quickly and continually assess, diagnose, plan, implement, and evaluate as the patient responds to the phases of the procedure and recovers from conscious sedation.

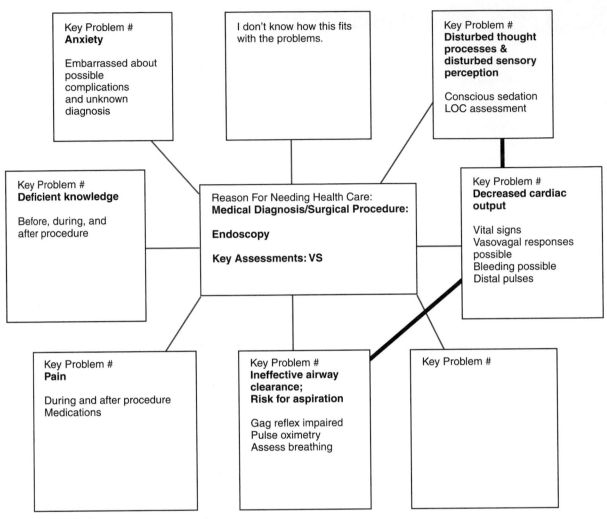

● Figure 5.3   Endoscopy procedure concept care map.

CHAPTER 5 SUMMARY

The focus of this chapter is on organizational strategies to promote the most efficient, productive, and safe clinical day. The chapter also focuses on using concept care maps as clinical organizational tools. Concept care maps are useful for organizing data in both inpatient and outpatient settings.

Concept care maps are used to organize and update patient assessment information, medications, IV fluids, treatments, and laboratory data when you arrive at the clinical unit. They are used to guide your patient assessments and evaluation of patient responses. They can be used to facilitate communications at the patient's bedside, in the medication area, and when you leave the unit for a break or at the end of the clinical day.

Step 5 of the concept care map is to take notes on patient responses to interventions, evaluate outcomes, and record an evaluative summary of the patient's progress toward outcome objectives. You must evaluate the patient's verbal and nonverbal behaviors, gather physical assessment data, and write notes in the patient response to interventions column of the nursing concept care map. These notes are the basis of documentation, which will be the focus of Chapter 7.

Reason for procedure	Recheck site where large polyp was removed and patient had large blood loss during removal procedure
Medical diagnosis	Polyps
Procedure	Colonoscopy with possible biopsy, polypectomy, or both
IV	No. 18 angiocatheter with 1000 cc 0.9% normal saline solution in right antecubital space
Vital signs	BP = 133/70 T = 95.8°F P = 68 R = 20
Height and weight	5'5" 120 lb
Review of systems	WNL all systems Sao₂ 99%
Psychosocial-cultural assessment	Catholic Married Anthem insurance Manager of a credit union During head-to-toe assessment, patient said she was nervous and afraid because of bad experience with bleeding when polyp was removed during the last procedure. Said she wanted to be completely knocked out for the procedure. Wanted a guarantee that she would not bleed like last time. Was visibly shaking.

● Figure 5.4   Patient data for endoscopy procedure.

 LEARNING ACTIVITIES

1. Preconference activity: Students should make comparisons with other students regarding medical and nursing diagnoses, concept care map diagrams, goals, objectives, and intervention lists. For example, if one student has a postoperative patient with a hip replacement and another student has a patient with a knee replacement, these students should compare concept care maps. The purpose of this exercise is to find similarities common to postoperative orthopedic patients and to become cognizant of individual differences among patients and treatment plans.

2. Devise, implement, and evaluate a plan of care on a real patient assignment in an inpatient or outpatient setting.

3. Class exercise: The purpose of this exercise is to compare step 5 patient responses in patients with similar diagnoses. Students should bring a

completed concept care map to class. Students assigned patients with similar diagnoses should form groups and review patient responses to nursing interventions. It should become apparent that, although patients may have similar medical and nursing diagnoses, the verbal and nonverbal responses listed in step 5 are unique, and progress toward outcomes varies from patient to patient.

4. Compare and contrast a concept care map developed for a diabetic inpatient with one developed for an outpatient undergoing endoscopy.

REFERENCES

1. Nursing's Social Policy Statement, ed 2. American Nurses Association, nurses-books.org, Washington, D.C., 2003.

2. Ibid.
3. Ibid.

6

INCLUDING PSYCHOSOCIAL-CULTURAL PROBLEMS IN THE CONCEPT CARE MAPS

OBJECTIVES

1. Identify crucial psycho-social-cultural characteristics to assess.
2. Describe how to perform the psycho-social-cultural assessment.
3. Integrate psycho-social-cultural diagnoses into the concept care map.
4. Develop goals, outcomes, and interventions for psycho-social-cultural diagnoses.
5. Record psycho-social-cultural patient responses.
6. Analyze relationships between psycho-social-cultural and physical diagnoses.

The purpose of this chapter is to expand on the assessment, diagnosis, planning, implementation, and evaluation of psycho-social-cultural problems. The patient profile database used in Chapter 2 focused on collection of relevant data the night before or day of clinical, primarily from patient records and a brief introduction to the patient and a brief discussion with the patient's staff nurse. Most of the information in patient records involves primarily physical data, with only a small amount of psycho-social-cultural data. Therefore, you will need to interact with patients directly to adequately assess their psycho-social-cultural problems.

You need time to interact with patients to establish therapeutic relationships with them. You also need to use therapeutic communication techniques to identify psycho-social-cultural problems and appropriate psycho-social-cultural nursing diagnoses and then develop appropriate goals, outcomes, and interventions as well as evaluation of patient responses. This chapter will focus on how to develop concept care maps for psycho-social-cultural problems.

Psycho-Social-Cultural and Developmental Assessment

Fundamental to the entire care planning and delivery process is your ability to communicate therapeutically and to form a therapeutic relationship. Therapeutic communication is critical to accurate psychosocial, cultural, and developmental assessment. It also forms the foundation of patient teaching. Assessing a patient's psychosocial, cultural, and developmental status is not the same as taking her history and her physical. In contrast to the history and the physical, the psycho-social-cultural assessment should not be based on direct questioning or interviewing.

Your objective is to develop rapport with your patients. Nurses must be able to have a comfortable conversation with a patient. The purpose of developing rapport is to help the patient relax enough to verbalize psycho-social-cultural concerns whenever they arise. Thus, the psycho-social-cultural assessment is integrated into and continues throughout basic patient care. You may have a number of physical goals to attain with your patient, such as improving skin integrity, decreasing pain, increasing cardiac output, improving gas exchange, and improving nutrition. As you work to attain these goals, you will need to work simultaneously on assessment and interventions for the patient's psycho-social-cultural problems.

Simultaneous assessment and intervention can be a difficult process to internalize and perform. You and your patient are both assessing and responding to each other minute to minute. As a professional nurse, your assessments and responses must be finely tuned to move the patient toward a healthier physical and psycho-social-cultural state (or a peaceful death), even while you are in the process of gathering data. You must learn the components of the psycho-social-cultural assessment very well so you know what to assess when interacting with your patients. Then, you must learn the appropriate psycho-social-cultural verbal and nonverbal responses and interventions. The psycho-social-cultural tool that appears in Figure 6.1 has been developed as a guide for student nurses to use during clinical interactions with patients.

The purpose of this tool is to serve as a general critical-thinking guide for assessing psycho-social-cultural problems. These problems can be very complex, perhaps even more complex than physical problems. There are numerous psycho-social-cultural nursing diagnoses, and it helps to have a foundational assessment tool as a general guideline. Therefore, the purpose of this assessment tool is to give you a starting point for collecting psycho-social-cultural data. It contains eight important components: the patient's current emotional state, life experiences, family, growth and development issues, relations with health-care providers, self-concept, culture, and gender. Each following numbered section corresponds with Figure 6.1.

1. Emotional State

Assessment of a patient's emotional state must be continuous. You should be consciously aware of the patient's mood by monitoring her verbal and nonverbal behaviors. Is the patient feeling anxious, fearful, sad, hopeless, lonely, or out of control? These are very common emotional reactions. Emotions affect a person's ability to concentrate and can interrupt thought processes. Without the ability to concentrate, it is very difficult for the patient or family to analyze problems carefully or to learn about self-care during a patient education session. Emotions also impair an individual's overall ability to communicate effectively.

One of the most important therapeutic techniques you need to learn and use is empathy. Empathy involves making clear to the patient that you have recognized the emotion the patient expresses. You must interpret the patient's emotional response correctly and then verbally communicate that understanding to the patient. It is important to acknowledge and accept emotions. For example, you can simply say "You seem sad." The purpose of empathy is to encourage ventilation by the patient as well as for you to demonstrate acceptance of the patient's emotions.

2. Life Experiences

Use therapeutic communication to assess and talk about changes in patient's social roles as a

Clinical Judgment _____

♦ 1. Emotional State
   Mood
   Body language
   Facial

♦ 2. Patient's Life Experience
   What are previous experiences with health care?

♦ 3. Family
   What is the mood of family members you meet?
   Are family members supportive?

♦ 4. Growth and Development–**Intimacy vs. Isolation**–Form an intimate bond with another person, growing independent of parents and managing a home, and taking on a career and becoming a responsible member of a community. **Generativity vs. Stagnation**–Remain productive with career, family and community social participation, and adjust to physical changes of middle age. **Ego integrity vs. Despair**–Content that they have played a meaningful part in the lives of those around them, adjust to changes in physical strength and find satisfactory living arrangements.
   How has this health problem interfered with growth and development?

♦ 5. Health Care Providers
   What is the patient/family current level of understanding of the health problem?
   Are they satisfied with the care they are receiving?

♦ 6. Self-esteem and Body Image
   What changes in physical appearance?
   What changes in activity?

♦ 7. Cultural Experiences
   Religious preference and practices?
   Favorite foods?
   Years lived in the region?
   Travel outside of the region?

♦ 8. Gender: What were the gender speech behaviors of the patient?

What communication techniques did you use with this patient? _____

➤ *Note: It is not appropriate to ask the patient direct questions as you would during a history. Information is obtained by observing verbal and nonverbal behaviors and making inferences as you and the patient work toward accomplishing objectives.*

● Figure 6.1   Psycho-social-cultural assessment tool clinical judgment.

result of health alterations. The role alterations may be temporary or permanent, but the change will cause concern for patients and significant others. Talk with your patient about the circumstances surrounding how he came to be in the health-care setting and his perception of his current situation. For example, with a hospitalized patient, determine how his or her life has changed as a result of hospitalization; find out who is at home and how everyone in the family is managing while this family member is hospi-

talized. Consider how the problem has interfered with the patient's lifestyle and the goals the patient was trying to accomplish at the time the problem occurred. Also consider the type of work the patient does and the type of leisure activities he enjoys.

3. Family and Significant Others

Social support is crucial to successful recovery. Take time to assess the ability of the patient's significant other to cope with the situation and to provide support for the patient. Family and friends commonly feel stress and strain when dealing with the patient's health problem and with the logistics of maintaining their home life and responsibilities.

4. Growth and Development

Assess growth and development tasks as appropriate to the patient's age. The stages of growth and development were described by Eric Erickson[1] and included in Chapter 2. Consider how the patient's health problem is interfering with his ability to perform appropriate growth and development tasks. For example, in young adulthood, tasks involve establishing intimacy and sexual roles, maintaining friendships, growing independent of parents, and establishing a career. A lengthy illness can severely disrupt all of these tasks.

5. Relations with Health-Care Providers

The nature of a patient's relationship with health-care providers is very important to assess. It is important to know whether the health-care providers and the patient have been able to establish a working relationship and to develop mutual goals. The first consideration is the patient's ability to communicate. Some patients with impaired cognitive functioning—such as those with Alzheimer's disease—probably will not be able to communicate effectively and make rational decisions. Thus, the family will be working closely with the health-care providers to discuss goals and outcomes.

Determine whether the patient and family understand the treatment regimen and whether they agree with and support it. Assess whether the patient and family have doubts or concerns about the plan. While providing care, look for evidence of clear or unclear communication between health-care providers and the patient or family. Stay alert to the level of understanding the patient and family have about the plan of care. You may want to ask the patient or a family member a general question such as, "What has the doctor been saying to you about your diabetes?" or "What have the nurses been teaching you about your diabetes?" After listening to the patient's answer, you can follow with a general probing question such as, "What do you think of all this?" Another good question to use to determine the patient's level of understanding for inpatient settings is, "Do you know when you are going home?" By staying alert and asking prudent questions, you can get a reasonable idea of the patient's and family's understanding of and feelings about the patient's problem.

Compliance is another issue that occurs in relationships between patients and health-care providers. Some patients and families may be noncompliant with or nonadherent to the treatment plan. The goals and outcomes between the health-care provider and patient or family may not be mutual. For example, a patient with a lung condition may refuse to stop smoking. Not all patients are going to be fully compliant with all aspects of the plan of care; they are diagnosed with *Impaired Adjustment*. First, you must determine if the patient understands what is wrong and has been given explanations about how to stop smoking. You must also determine if the patient has the means by which to implement a smoking cessation plan if he decides he wants to do so. Ultimately, it is the patient's decision to agree or not to agree with any aspect of a therapeutic regimen.

Finally, another common relational problem involves turmoil over deciding what to do. The patient and family may have several health-care options from which they need to choose. For example, should a grandmother go to a nursing home, or should she move in with one of her children? Should the patient undergo chemotherapy for cancer? Health-care providers commonly guide patients in solving problems, especially as they examine their options. But it is the patient's and family's right to select the option that best suits them.

6. Self-Esteem and Body Image

It is important to assess the patient's self-concept pertaining to self-esteem and body image. Self-esteem is the value that people place on themselves. Because it is not appropriate to ask, "How is your self-esteem today?" you will need to try to infer it from the patient's body language, tone of voice, and words. As you interact with a patient, you can get clues to a person's sense of self-esteem by paying attention to expressions of feeling worthwhile or useless. People with high self-esteem usually can openly and honestly express what they think and feel. Even though patients have health problems, those with high self-esteem typically believe they are likable, are capable of handling the challenge of the health problem, and are effective in dealing with problems. According to Satir,[2] patients with low self-esteem placate, blame, compute, or distract. The placater tries to do whatever someone else says, not because she wants to but because she wants the other person to like her and to not be mad at her. The blamer reacts to problems by yelling and giving orders. Beneath this exterior the person believes nobody loves or cares for her. The computer believes that showing emotions is a sign of weakness; this person lives by logic and rationalizations, although he feels very vulnerable. The distracter uses disruptions to get attention, has difficulty focusing on the issues at hand, and believes that no one cares about him. For a discussion of effective therapeutic communication with patients with low self-esteem, read Chapter 5, "Breaking Through Barriers to Successful Communication" in Schuster, *Communication: The Key to the Therapeutic Relationship.*

Closely linked to self-esteem is body image. Body image refers to a person's feelings and attitudes toward the physical body. If a person feels good about how he looks, it improves his self-esteem. If he feels bad about how he looks, it worsens his self-esteem. Many illnesses and the aging process alter the structure and functioning of the physical body, and body image disturbances result. Scars, deformities, amputations, weight gain or loss, and hair loss are examples of *Disturbed Body Image.* They may cause patients to be confused about how they perceive themselves. It takes time to integrate and accommodate changes in physical structure and function.

7. Cultural Experiences

It is important to assess the patient's cultural beliefs and practices. Cultural issues affect the plan of care. Many people are of mixed cultures; families have lived in the United States for generations. Everyone has beliefs and behaviors that have been passed down, although the origins of the beliefs and behaviors may not be known. Purnell's[3] model will be used as a guide for assessment of cultural experiences.

Purnell's model for cultural competence is an excellent tool for cultural assessment. The components of this model that are most relevant to cultural assessments of patients and their families are outlined in Box 6.1 and include heritage,

---

Box 6.1   COMPONENTS OF PURNELL'S MODEL FOR ASSESSMENT OF CULTURE

▶ Heritage
▶ Communication
▶ Family roles and organization
▶ Biocultural ecology
▶ High-risk behaviors
▶ Nutrition
▶ Pregnancy and childbearing
▶ Death rituals
▶ Spirituality
▶ Health-seeking beliefs and behaviors
▶ Culture of health-care practitioners
▶ Cultural workforce issues

communication, family roles and organization, biocultural ecology, high-risk behaviors, nutrition, pregnancy and childbearing, death rituals, spirituality, health-seeking beliefs and behaviors, the culture of health-care practitioners, and cultural workforce issues.

Heritage

A person's country of origin commonly plays an important role in the development of her ideas and beliefs. For everyone, except for Native Americans, it is especially important to consider why the person, family, or cultural group migrated to the United States. Most emigrate in hopes of a better life, but it may help you to know a more specific motivating factor. For example, migration may have resulted from political oppression, religious persecution, lack of job opportunities, or a natural disaster. Past economic and political experiences directly affect the individual's ideologies. It is important to consider the patient's and family's extent of orientation to their new culture and their familiarity with the U.S. health-care system and providers.

Communication

In addition to the influence of language barriers on communication, also consider whether the patient feels comfortable sharing his thoughts and feelings. Cultural communication involves the amount of touch that is acceptable, personal space expected, and eye contact deemed appropriate and the types and meanings of facial expressions used and body language displayed. Temporal relationships are also important to understand because the expectations regarding punctuality vary among cultures. In addition, there are differing expectations regarding how to properly address people to maintain respect.

Family Roles and Organization

It is important to determine the dominant member of the household: the person in the family who is the spokesperson and decision maker. In addition, the patient's nuclear family, extended family, and living space are important considerations in the plan of care, particularly with respect to the level of support the family gives to

the member who needs health care. If family members cannot cope with the problem, other arrangements will need to be made.

Biocultural Ecology

Cultural groups have specific genetic, physical, and biological characteristics, such as skin color, bone structure, and metabolism. These characteristics are noted in the general physical screening examinations. Health-care providers need to screen for specific health problems in different cultural groups because some diseases are genetically and environmentally transmitted. For example, sickle cell disease, diabetes, and malaria occur with increased prevalence in particular ethnic groups. This information is routinely available on patient records and is part of the basic history screening examination.

High-Risk Behaviors

High-risk behaviors include the use of tobacco, alcohol, and recreational drugs; participation in high-risk physical activities; and lack of adherence to important health-safety practices. Behaviors may vary with the cultural group and must be explored with each patient. Assessment of high-risk behaviors is typically part of the general screening health history.

Nutrition

A patient's diet is integral to many health problems and must be a topic of assessment. It is important that you become aware of the basic ingredients of native food dishes and preparation practices to provide culturally competent dietary counseling. Each cultural group has food preferences. The goal of dietary counseling is to select healthy foods from within the culturally preferred choices, not to require the patient to follow a typical American diet as part of the plan of care. Cultural meaning may be attached to foods that the patient eats or avoids. Food is often associated with cultural rituals.

Pregnancy and Childbearing Practices

Patients' beliefs and practices regarding fertility, birth control, pregnancy, birthing, and postpartum care vary widely, based in part on cultural background. For example, selection of birth control methods, roles of men in childbirth, positions for delivering a baby, and preferred types of health practitioners (male or female, midwife or obstetrician) commonly vary among people of different cultural groups.

Death Rituals

It is important to identify culturally specific death rituals and mourning practices. Each culture has its own view of death, dying, and the afterlife. One of the goals of nursing a dying patient is to provide the means for a peaceful death, and that can be accomplished only if you know the person's and family's death rituals. For example, a Catholic patient may want a priest to administer last rites, and a Muslim patient may want the bed positioned to face Mecca.

Spirituality

It is important to assess the dominant religion of an ethnic group and to be aware of the patient's and family's use of activities such as prayer or meditation as a source of comfort. You should know how to contact the patient's religious leaders if the patient or family so desires. Spirituality does not always involve a specific religion: it involves beliefs about the meaning and purposes of life. The patient's and family's spirituality may be a source of emotional strength and sustenance through trying health-care situations.

Health-Seeking Beliefs and Behaviors

It is important to assess the predominant beliefs influencing a patient's health-care practices. Practices involve care of the sick, health promotion, and prevention. Cultures vary in their beliefs about pain, mental and physical handicaps, and chronic illness. Determine who will assume responsibility for care of the sick and the role of health insurance in the culture. Included in this category are folklore practices that influence health behaviors. For example, blood transfusions or implantation of electrical devices may not be acceptable to a cultural group, although these are common medical practices.

Culture of the Health-Care Practitioners

When the health professional and patient are from different cultures, there may be a lack of trust if either person considers the other to be an outsider. The gender and age of the health-care provider are also important to consider in providing culturally competent care. The status accorded health-care providers and their advice varies among cultures.

Cultural Workforce Issues

As a nurse, you will almost certainly work in a multicultural environment. Patients and health-care providers come from a variety of cultural backgrounds. The primary factors related to work include language barriers, amount of assimilation, and autonomy issues. For example, difficulties may arise in the workplace from differing values placed on timeliness and punctuality, learning styles, personality styles, and levels of assertiveness. As you develop concept care maps for patients and families, learn to be culturally sensitive not only to patients and their families but also to other health-care providers from different cultural backgrounds.

It is impossible to know the beliefs and practices of every culture, but health-care providers intent on providing culturally competent care continue to learn through traveling, reading, and attending events held by local ethnic and cultural organizations as well as drawing on the expertise of colleagues. Health-care providers need to learn to conduct a cultural assessment effectively and then analyze and solve health-care problems of patients and their family members from the perspective of the patient's cultural group. Culturally competent health-care professionals must be highly proficient in therapeutic communication.

Of special significance is that health-care providers refrain from making judgments about cultural behaviors and practices they deem strange or "wrong." There are many ways to attain a mutual goal; to be philosophical, there are many paths to the same destination. Health-care providers must be resourceful and creative, and they should tailor interventions to suit the patient's culture. They must respect differences and appreciate the inherent worth of diverse cultures. The first step in becoming culturally competent is to become aware of your own values, attitudes, and beliefs. The learning activities at the end of the chapter are designed to teach you about your own ethnic background.

8. Gender

Gender differences in communication are partially derived from cultural background. Tannen's[4] work on gender differences in styles of communication will help guide your assessment. Tannen's views on gender differences may help you respond appropriately to differing styles of speech in male and female patients. Communication patterns are culturally ingrained, although there may also be a biological basis for gender differences in communication. Tannen's research suggests that women speak, at least in part, to promote intimacy and to form communal connections, whereas men in their speech are more likely to focus on hierarchy, status attainment, and demonstration of status. As a nurse, you must learn to respond to patients based on the speech patterns you discern. General characteristics of male and female speech patterns are listed in Table 6.1. You may need to alter your communication patterns to suit the gender of your patient. For a more detailed discussion of how to accomplish this goal and what nursing implications may arise, read Chapter 2, "Gender Differences in Communication" of Schuster, *Communication: The Key to the Therapeutic Relationship*.[5]

The psycho-social-cultural assessment tool is to be used as a guide for collecting data. Bring this guide to clinical to assist you in the development of the psycho-social-cultural components of the concept care map. The guide entails eight basic categories of characteristics to assess as you work with the patient and family. Be aware, however, that more in-depth assessment of a particular area may be needed, depending on the situation. A vast amount of literature exists on each of the components of the psycho-social-cultural assessment guide. The guide barely scratches the surface of available knowledge, but it does provide a starting point for data collection.

Developing and Integrating the Psycho-Social-Cultural Aspects of the Concept Care Map

Throughout the clinical day, you will assess, diagnose, plan, implement, and evaluate psycho-social-cultural problems. In this section, we will develop a clinical case study in detail to illustrate how you can integrate psycho-social-cultural data into your plan of care. A patient with breast cancer and a mastectomy will be used to illustrate this process.

Start with the initial patient profile database for the mastectomy patient who was presented in Chapter 3. The patient profile database is reproduced for you in Figure 6.2. A student nurse collected this information on the day of surgery in preparation for care of the patient on the first postoperative day. A basic "sloppy copy" concept care map for steps 1 to 3 could look like what appears in Figure 6.3. Remember that concept care maps vary in appearance, but all the essential data are there.

This care map would need to be updated on arrival to the unit for the latest information on the patient as described in Chapter 5. As you can see, the map includes data regarding physical pathology and physical assessment, medications, treatments, and laboratory results. Psycho-social-cultural problems are present but not known in detail. The student nurse could infer that the patient may have some form of depression because she is taking the drug Zoloft (ser-

Table 6.1 Traditional Gender Differences in Communication	
Female	*Male*
Rapport talk	Report talk
Less adversarial	More adversarial
Cooperative overlapper	Talks alone
Listener	Information provider
Personal storytelling	Storytelling of human contests
Uses tag questions	Does not use tag questions
Conversational rituals:	Conversational rituals:
"I'm sorry"	Joking
"Thanks"	Teasing
	Sarcasm

Student Name: **MAB**

1) Date of Care: **12/24**	2) Patient Initials: **AL**	3) Age: **78** (face sheet)	3) Growth and Development **Ego integrity vs. Despair**	4) Gender: **F** (face sheet)	5) Admission Date: (face sheet) **12/3**

6) Reason for hospitalization (face sheet): Describe reason for hospitalization: (expand on back of page) *Medical Dx:* **Breast Cancer** *Pathophysiology:* *All signs and symptoms: Highlight those your patient exhibits*	7) Chronic illnesses (physician's history and physical notes in chart; nursing intake assessment and Kardex) **NIDDM** **Hypertension** **MI 1994**
8) Surgical procedures (consent forms and Kardex): Describe surgical procedure (expand on back of page) Name of surgical procedure: **Mastectomy** *Describe surgery:* **Right modified radical mastectomy**	

9) ADVANCE DIRECTIVES (NURSE'S ADMISSION ASSESSMENTS):

Living will: ☐ Yes ☐ No	Power of attorney: ☐ Yes ☐ No	Do not resuscitate (DNR) order (Kardex): ☐ Yes ☐ No

10) LABORATORY DATA:

Test	Normal Values	Admission 12/3	Date/Time 12/4	Date/Time	Reason for Abnormal Values
White blood cells (WBCs)		5.6	4.8		
Red blood cells (RBCs)					
Hemoglobin (Hgb)		11.2	11		
Hematocrit (Hct)		33.2	33.1		
Platelets		259,000			
Prothrombin time (PT)					
International normalized ratio (INR)					
Activated partial thromboplastin time (Aptt)					
Sodium Na					
Potassium K		2.8	2.8		
Chloride Cl					
Glucose (FBS/BS)		230	235		
Hemoglobin A1C					
Cholesterol					
Blood Urea Nitrogen (BUN)					
Creatinine					
Urine analysis (UA)					
Pre-albumin					
Albumin					
Calcium Ca					
Phosphate					
Bilirubin					
Alkaline phosphatase					
SGOT-Serum glutamic-oxyloacetic transaminase					
AST-Serum glutamic pyruvic transaminase					
CK					
CK MB					
Troponin					
B-natriuretic peptide BNP					
pH					
pCO_2					
pO_2					
HCO_3					

11) DIAGNOSTIC TESTS

Chest x-ray:	EKG:	Other abnormal reports:
Sputum or Blood Culture:	Other:	Other:

12) MEDICATIONS   List medications and times of administration (medication administration record and check the drawer in the carts for spelling). Include over-the- counter (OTC) products/herbal medicines.

Times Due	1000	0800	1000	1000
Brand Name		Lasix	Tenormin	Zoloft
Generic Name	heparin	furosemide	atenolol	sertraline
Dose	5000U	40mg	25mg	25mg
Administration Route	sq	po	po	po
Classification				
Action				
Reason This Patient is Receiving				
Pharmacokinetics	O P D 1/2 M E	O P D 1/2 M E	O P D 1/2 M E	O P D 1/2 M E
Contraindications				
Major Adverse Side Effects				
Nursing Implications				
Pt/Family Teaching				

Developed by P. Testa, YSU

Times Due	1000	1000	1000	q4h pm
Brand Name	Lanoxin	Ecotrin	K-dur	Darvocet N-100
Generic Name	digoxin	aspirin	KCl	Propoxyphene Acetaminophen
Dose	01.25mg	1 tablet	20mg	100mg/650mg
Administration Route	po	po	po	po
Classification				
Action				
Reason This Patient is Receiving				
Pharmacokinetics	O P D 1/2 M E	O P D 1/2 M E	O P D 1/2 M E	O P D 1/2 M E
Contraindications				
Major Adverse Side Effects				
Nursing Implications				
Pt/Family Teaching				

Developed by P. Testa, YSU

ALLERGIES/PAINS

13) Allergies: **NKA** Type of Reaction: (medication administration record):	14) When was the last time pain medication given? (medication administration record) **Darvocet 6am (getting it sporadically)**
14) Where is the pain? **surgical incision** (nurse's notes)	14) How much pain is the patient in on a scale from 0-10? (nurse's notes, flow sheet): **5, confusion makes it unreliable**

TREATMENTS

15) List Treatments (Kardex): Rationale for treatments:
Dressing changes—sterile gauze & surgical bra, change qam
Ice to incision
Ted hose
IS q2h while awake
C&DB q2h while awake
I and O, & record q1h x 2

16) Support services (Kardex) What do support services provide for the patient?

17) What does the consultant do for the patient?:

18) DIET/FLUIDS

| Type of Diet (Kardex): **1800 ADA** | Restrictions (Kardex): | Gag reflex intact: ☐Yes ☐No | Appetite: ☐Good ☐Fair ☒Poor | Breakfast **Eating Jello and tea only** | Lunch ___ % | Dinner ___ % |

What type of diet is this?:

What types of foods are included in this diet and what foods should be avoided?:

Circle Those Problems That Apply:

| **Prior 24 hours** Fluid intake: (Oral & IV) **2100** Fluid output **1700** (flow sheet) | • Problems: swallowing, chewing, dentures (nurse's notes) • Needs assistance with feeding (nurse's notes) • Nausea or vomiting (nurse's notes) • Overhydrated or dehydrated (evaluate total intake and output on flow sheet |
| Tube feedings: Type and rate (Kardex) | • Belching: • Other: _____ **Dentures and Needs Assistance Eating** |

19) INTRAVENOUS FLUIDS (IV therapy record)

| Type and Rate: **LR with 20 KCl 100/h** | IV dressing dry, no edema, redness of site: ☒Yes ☐No | Other: |

20) ELIMINATION (flow sheet)

| Last bowel movement: **None since surgery** | Foley/condom catheter: ☐Yes ☒No |

Circle Those Problems That Apply:

• Bowel: constipation diarrhea flatus incontinence belching
• Urinary: hesitancy frequency burning incontinence odor
• Other: _____
• What is causing the problem in elimination? _____

21) ACTIVITY (Kardex, flow sheet)

| Ability to walk (gait): | Type of activity orders: **up as tolerated** | Use of assistance devices: cane, walker, crutches, prosthesis: | Falls-risk assessment rating: **7 high** |
| No. of side rails required (flow sheet) **4** | Restraints (flow sheet): ☒Yes ☐No **vest, wrist** | Weakness ☒Yes ☐No | Trouble sleeping (nurse's notes): ☒Yes ☐No |

What does activity order mean?: _____
Why isn't the patient up ad lib?: _____
Would the problem cause weakness?: _____

PHYSICAL ASSESSMENT DATA

| 22) BP (flow sheet): **137/72** **152/100** | 2) TPR (flow sheet): **97-52-20** **97.8-80-20** | 23) Height: __5'5"__ Weight: __190#__ (nursing intake assessments) |

24) NEUROLOGICAL/MENTAL STATUS:

| LOC: alert and oriented to person, place, time (A&O x 3) confused, etc. **Alert & oriented to person only, became confused evening after surgery** | Speech: clear, appropriate/inappropriate **inappropriate** |
| Pupils: PERRLA | Sensory deficits for vision/hearing/taste/ smell **glasses** |

25) MUSCULOSKELETAL STATUS:

Bones, joints, muscles (fractures, contractures, arthritis, spinal curvatures, etc):	Extremity (temperature, edema (pitting vs. nonpitting) & sensation)
Motor: ROM x 4 extremities	
Ted hose/plexi pulses/compression devices: type:	Casts, splint, collar, brace:

26) CARDIOVASCULAR SYSTEM:

Pulses (radial, pedal) (to touch or with Doppler):	Capillary refill (<3s): ☐ Yes ☐ No	
Neck vein (distention):	Sounds: S1, S2, regular, irregular: Apical rate: **80**	Any chest pain:

27) RESPIRATORY SYSTEM:

Depth, rate, rhythm: **20**	Use of accessory muscles:	Cyanosis:	Sputum color, amount:	Cough: productive nonproductive	Breath sounds: clear, rales, wheezes **Clear, decreased in bases**
Use of oxygen: nasal cannula, mask, trach collar:	Flow rate of oxygen:	Oxygen humidification: ☐ Yes ☐ No		Pulse oximeter: _____ % oxygen saturation	Smoking: ☐ Yes ☐ No

28) GASTROINTESTINAL SYSTEM

Abdominal pain, tenderness, guarding; distention, soft, firm: **Soft & nondistended**	Bowel sounds x 4 quadrants: **Active 4 quads**	NG tube: describe drainage
Ostomy: describe stoma site and stools:	Other:	

29) SKIN AND WOUNDS:

Color, turgor: **Pink, poor turgor**	Rash, bruises: **Dry and chapped**	Describe wounds (size, locations): **Red & edematous**	Edges approximated: ☒ Yes ☐ No	Type of wound drains: **JP #1 25 ml** **JP #2 100 ml**
Characteristics of drainage: **serosanguineous**	Dressings (clean, dry, intact): **Clean, dry, intact**	Sutures, staples, steri-strips, other:	Risk for pressure ulcer assessment rating:	Other:

30) EYES, EARS, NOSE, THROAT (EENT):

Eyes: redness, drainage, edema, ptosis	Ears: drainage	Nose: redness, drainage, edema	Throat: sore

Psychosocial and Cultural Assessment

31) Religious preference (face sheet) **Catholic**	32) Marital status (face sheet) **Widowed**	33) Health care benefits and insurance (face sheet): **Medicare**
34) Occupation (face sheet) **Housewife**	35) Emotional state (nurse's notes) **Anxious, wants to go home, very talkative, does not respond to questions appropriately**	

● Figure 6.2 Patient profile database: A surgical patient with a mastectomy.

traline) and because the removal of a breast is disfiguring and may influence her most intimate relationships. Therefore, there is evidence to support the nursing diagnoses of *Disturbed Body Image* and *Chronic Sorrow*. There is little assessment information to support these diagnoses, so the nurse must continue the assessment during the clinical day. As the nurse continues to interact with the patient, she is able to do a more thorough continuation of the psycho-social-cultural assessment and gain more information regarding the cultural and developmental factors that will necessitate modification of the basic concept care map.

After the care map has been updated as described in Chapter 5, the student nurse will

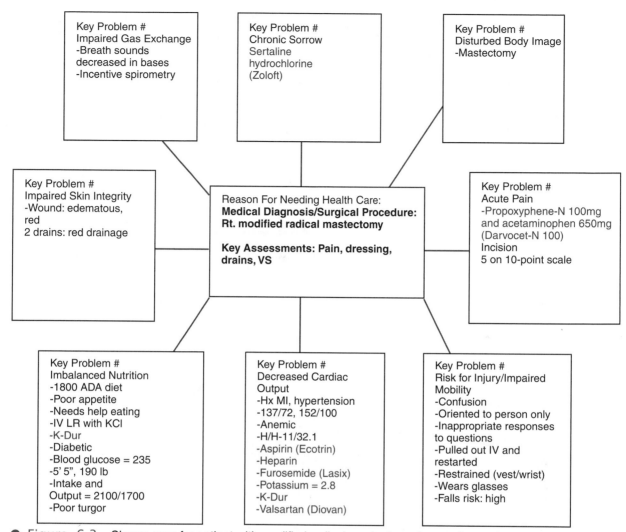

Key Problem #
Impaired Gas Exchange
-Breath sounds decreased in bases
-Incentive spirometry

Key Problem #
Chronic Sorrow
Sertaline hydrochlorine (Zoloft)

Key Problem #
Disturbed Body Image
-Mastectomy

Key Problem #
Impaired Skin Integrity
-Wound: edematous, red
2 drains: red drainage

Reason For Needing Health Care:
**Medical Diagnosis/Surgical Procedure:
Rt. modified radical mastectomy**

Key Assessments: Pain, dressing, drains, VS

Key Problem #
Acute Pain
-Propoxyphene-N 100mg and acetaminophen 650mg (Darvocet-N 100)
Incision
5 on 10-point scale

Key Problem #
Imbalanced Nutrition
-1800 ADA diet
-Poor appetite
-Needs help eating
-IV LR with KCl
-K-Dur
-Diabetic
-Blood glucose = 235
-5' 5", 190 lb
-Intake and Output = 2100/1700
-Poor turgor

Key Problem #
Decreased Cardiac Output
-Hx MI, hypertension
-137/72, 152/100
-Anemic
-H/H-11/32.1
-Aspirin (Ecotrin)
-Heparin
-Furosemide (Lasix)
-Potassium = 2.8
-K-Dur
-Valsartan (Diovan)

Key Problem #
Risk for Injury/Impaired Mobility
-Confusion
-Oriented to person only
-Inappropriate responses to questions
-Pulled out IV and restarted
-Restrained (vest/wrist)
-Wears glasses
-Falls risk: high

● Figure 6.3   Sloppy copy for patient with modified radical mastectomy (preconference); carry in pocket at all times!

begin the initial key-assessments by checking the patient's vital signs, pain levels, and dressing. *Confusion* is a critical safety concern that is a priority assessment. Imagine that the student nurse goes into the patient's room and says hello. The patient is confused and asks, "Where am I? Where is my son?" The patient begins to cry and says, "I want to go home." The student nurse may infer that the patient is probably anxious and sad because she is confused and tearful about where she is and who the nurse is. The student may infer that the patient may also feel very lonely and out of control. The student introduces herself, tells the patient where she is, takes the patient's hand, gives the patient some tissues, and explains quietly and calmly that she needs to check the blood pressure and dressing, and that she is going to take care of her. The student asks if the patient is hurting anywhere, and the patient responds, "No, I want my son Bobby." The student nurse tells the patient that she will try to find Bobby, and then she explains that she needs to check with the staff nurse and her faculty and that she will return very soon.

After leaving the room, the student nurse's initial impressions were as follows: this patient is anxious; she wants to go home, she is crying, and she misses her son. She also has acute confusion and is oriented only to her name. The student nurse adds these impressions to the concept care map, as shown in Figure 6.4. It was originally included with the diagnosis of *Risk for Injury*, but as soon as the student talked to the patient, it was clearly evident that her *Confusion* was a major nursing diagnosis and needed special consideration.

The student nurse then discusses the situation with her faculty, who validates the diagnoses. Recognizing relationships between psycho-

social-cultural diagnoses is very important. For example, as anxiety increases, confusion would also probably increase. It is important to recognize that physical problems affect and are interconnected with psycho-social-cultural problems and vice versa. Humans respond in a holistic manner to health problems. Lines are drawn (see Fig. 6.4) to show relationships among the patient's problems.

Before writing outcomes and interventions, you need to take note of how the student nurse

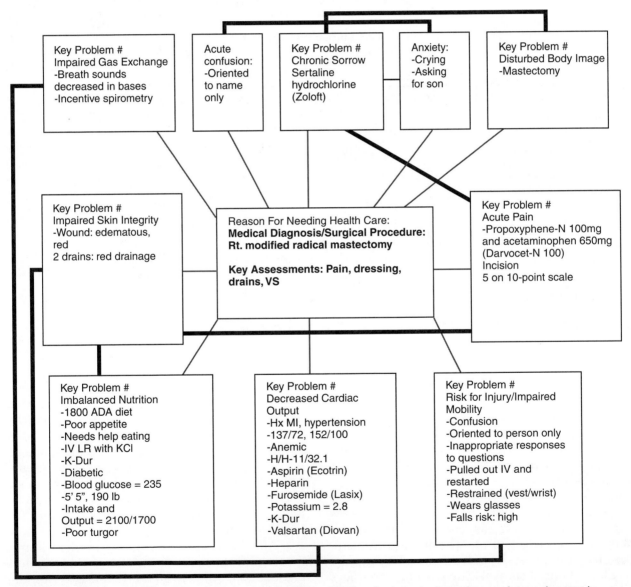

● Figure 6.4   Revised sloppy copy for patient with modified radical mastectomy (preconference); carry in pocket at all times!

intervened immediately when he recognized a problem in the above scenario. What therapeutic communication interventions were used by the nurse in the scenario above?

Next, plan interventions to help decrease *Anxiety* and *Confusion*. The intervention list has been started for you, along with the goals and outcomes, in Figure 6.5. It is important to understand that psycho-social-cultural interventions are purposeful therapeutic communication techniques that are performed while continuing the assessment. As you read the continuation of the scenario, identify the therapeutic communication techniques used by the student nurse as she continued the psycho-social-cultural assessment along with providing physical care.

The student nurse checks with the staff nurse, who says the patient's son Bobby is coming in soon and that he just called in to check on her. Bobby states that his mother has not been confused at home and that he cannot understand why this is happening now. The staff nurse assures Bobby that the doctors were trying to determine the cause of the confusion and that sometimes patients react in such a manner to anesthetics or medications. He also assures Bobby that his mother was being watched carefully. The staff nurse asked Bobby to bring in a family picture or some other object to help reorient his mother.

The student nurse goes back to the patient to finish her assessment and help the patient with breakfast. She makes small talk as she does the physical assessment, using distraction as the therapeutic technique, talking about the patient's pretty blue robe that matches her blue eyes. The patient says that her daughter bought her the robe for her birthday. The patient's son comes in, and she brightens when she sees him and asks him to take her home.

The student nurse continues the psycho-social-cultural assessment with the patient's son present and asks with whom the patient lives. Bobby explains that he and his son live with his mother, who cooks and cleans and takes care of them. He also explains that she is very active with the ladies guild of St. Joseph's Catholic Church. He says that he wants to get her home as soon as possible. He brought in a school picture of his 15-year-old son and puts it on the night stand. The student nurse tells the patient

what a handsome grandson she has, and the patient smiles.

The patient's son asks if the doctor has been in yet because he wants to talk about why his mother was confused. The student nurse says she will go to page the doctor. When she returns to the room, she says the doctor will arrive shortly.

Based on these interactions, can you identify the important points of exchange between the student nurse and the patient's son that are components of the psycho-social-cultural assessment tool in Figure 6.1?

The student nurse next goes over the basic problems and what she intends to do to correct the problems with both the patient and the patient's son. The patient and her son must know the goals and expected outcomes for the day. As the student nurse goes over the plan, she can further assess cultural issues. For example, the student may tell the patient and family that eating foods to promote wound healing is important. She asks what kinds of foods the patient likes to eat and finds out that the patient prefers the Italian food of her heritage as well as sweets of all kinds.

The student nurse discusses the need to keep the patient safe from falls and discusses her activity limitations and the use of restraints for safety. She also discusses the need to monitor vital signs and the care of the wound. In addition, the student discusses the need to improve oxygenation and to control pain.

The physician comes in and says that the patient may be reacting to the anesthetic and that her electrolytes are a little off and are being corrected. The physician also says that the patient's wound is healing as anticipated. The son explains that he wants to take his mother home as soon as possible and that he and his sister (who lives next door) would take care of her at home. He believes that once she gets back to her own home his mother will not be as confused. The physician wants to keep the patient in the hospital for just another day to regulate her electrolytes and to monitor her. The son agrees.

Recording Patient Responses

Patient responses to psychosocial and cultural issues should be recorded across from the nursing interventions in the same manner as

Problem # ___ : Acute Anxiety
General Goal: **Decreased Anxiety**

Predicted Behavioral Outcome Objective (s): The patient will…Talk about concerns, smile, rest peacefully… on the day of care.

Nursing Interventions   Patient Responses to Interventions

1. Assess anxiety   1. _____
2. Use therapeutic communication   2. _____
3. Use distraction   3. _____
4. _____   4. _____
5. _____   5. _____
6. _____   6. _____
7. _____   7. _____
8. _____   8. _____

Evaluation: Summarize patient progress toward outcome objectives:
_____
_____

Problem #_____ : Confusion
General Goal: **Decreased Confusion**

Predicted Behavioral Outcome Objective (s): The patient will…not have injuries, and state why she is in the hospital… on the day of care.

Nursing Interventions   Patient Responses to Interventions

1. Assess confusion   1. _____
2. Use reality orientation   2. _____
3. Use familiar objects   3. _____
4. _____   4. _____
5. _____   5. _____
6. _____   6. _____
7. _____   7. _____
8. _____   8. _____

Evaluation: Summarize patient progress toward outcome objectives:
_____
_____

● Figure 6.5   Psychosocial nursing diagnoses, goals, objectives, interventions, and responses.

described in Chapter 5. Remember to notice the patient's verbal and nonverbal behaviors. For example, how does the patient respond to touch? Does she withdraw or smile? Also, write your impressions about the patient's progress toward or away from objectives. Did the patient's responses lead you to conclude that she was talking about her concerns? Was she able to state where she was and why she was there? Record possible patient responses in the Patient Responses to Interventions column in Figure 6.5.

CHAPTER 6 SUMMARY

Psycho-social-cultural problems are often not known until you have face-to-face interactions with a patient. The focus of the initial concept care map is generally on physical information and treatments because, typically, only a small amount of psycho-social-cultural information is available in patient records. The bulk of the information concerns physical pathology problems, medications, treatments, and laboratory results.

Assessment of a person's psychosocial and cultural development should be integrated throughout the time you work with the patient. Information collection is more informal than it is during a history and physical, and it should not be done through direct questioning and interviewing. It is accomplished by observing nonverbal behaviors, responses to touch, and facial mannerisms and having conversations with patients and family members.

There are eight major areas on which to focus when doing the psycho-social-cultural assessment, summarized in Box 6.2. The current emotional state assessment should be done continually and interventions performed as needed to promote emotional relaxation and comfort. Previous life experiences and how the problem disrupts the patient's lifestyle are important to consider, along with the effects of the problems on the family and significant others. Growth and development is disrupted by illness and interferes with a person's ability to accomplish expected tasks of growth and development. Self-esteem and body image can be altered when a health condition affects the patient's feelings of worth and feelings about their physical body. Cultural assessment involves the consideration of heritage, communication patterns, family roles and organization, biocultural ecology, high-risk behaviors, nutrition, pregnancy and childbearing practices, death rituals, spirituality, and health-seeking behaviors. Gender differences may result in differences in styles of speech.

It is crucial for you to understand the relationship between psycho-social-cultural problems and physical problems. Psycho-social-cultural problems affect how physical problems are manifested and treated and vice versa. The concept care map serves to illustrate these relationships. You can demonstrate your knowledge of the integration of physical and psychosocial diagnoses by drawing lines to show relationships on concept care maps. The goals, outcomes, interventions, and responses involving psycho-social-cultural problems are written in the same format as described in previous chapters for physical problems.

Another important point to be made is that both physical and psycho-social-cultural assessments are ongoing throughout the clinical day. Changes in goals, outcomes, and interventions sometimes occur on a minute-to-minute basis based on new assessment information or a new evaluation of patient responses. The aim is to provide comprehensive holistic care.

LEARNING ACTIVITIES

1. In class, form groups of three or four, and relate examples of therapeutic communication techniques you would use to develop a therapeutic relationship with a patient. For example, empathy is a key therapeutic communication technique. What would you say to show empathy? Other therapeutic communication techniques include supportive touch, humor, problem solving, decision making, increasing patient self-esteem, increasing patient assertiveness, positive reinforcement, encouragement, distraction, reality orientation, reminiscing, anticipatory guidance, and showing pos-

---

Box 6.2   A SUMMARY OF PSYCHO-SOCIAL-CULTURAL ASSESSMENT GUIDELINES

1. **Current Emotional State**
   Use therapeutic communication to do an emotional assessment, and find out the mood of the patient.

2. **Life Experiences**
   Use therapeutic communication to talk with your patient about the circumstances surrounding the need for health care and about the patient's perception of the current situation. How has life changed as a result of the problem? How has this problem interfered with the goals that the patient was trying to accomplish?

3. **Family**
   How are family members coping with the situation? Are family members supportive? Who is performing the roles the patient cannot because of the health problem?

4. **Growth and Development**
   What are the growth and developmental tasks relevant to the age of the patient? How has this health problem interfered with accomplishing growth and developmental tasks?

5. **Relations With Health-Care Providers**
   What has the physician and other members of the health-care team been saying to the patient and family? When are they going home (if applicable)? The aim is to determine the patient's cur-

rent understanding of the problem. In addition, what type of relationship does the patient have with health-care providers? Are they able and willing to follow directions for treatments (compliance)?

6. **Self-Concept**
   As you talk with the patient, what inferences can be made regarding self-esteem and body image as a result of the patient's health problems and situation? Does the patient appear to have confidence in her ability to care for herself, or does she have doubts and concerns? How accepting is she of the current situation?

7. **Culture**
   As you talk with the patient, assess gender and cultural beliefs and practices that are applicable to the current health-care situation. Key areas of assessment include responses to touch, personal space, eye contact, facial expressions, and body language. Determine the dominant family members and which family members have responsibility for health care. In addition, consider nutritional implications, spirituality, and cultural responses to pain.

8. **Gender**
   What are the gender speech patterns present in the situation?

---

itive regard. These techniques were reviewed in Chapter 4. Discuss the patient's specific verbal and nonverbal responses to the techniques. Write them on the board.

2. To evaluate your own cultural background, do the mini cultural assessment in Figure 6.6 at the end of this section. Get together in small groups to compare responses with classmates.

3. In class, form groups of three or four, and relate clinical examples of psycho-social-cultural problems that you have encountered in your experiences as nursing students. Give an example to fit each of the categories of the psychosocial, cultural, and developmental assessment guidelines. Give examples of alterations in emotional state, patient's life experiences, family, growth and development, relations with health-care providers, self-esteem, body image, culture, and gender. Elect a spokesperson to share examples with the entire class.

4. Practice developing psycho-social-cultural nursing diagnoses answering the following questions:

For each of these feelings, what is the psycho-social-cultural nursing diagnosis, and what are the verbal and nonverbal behaviors that indicate each emotion?

Anxious

Nursing diagnosis_____

Verbal_____

Nonverbal_____

Fearful

Nursing diagnosis_____

Verbal_____

Nonverbal_____

Sad

Nursing diagnosis_____

Verbal_____

Nonverbal_____

Hopeless

Nursing diagnosis_____

Verbal_____

Nonverbal_____

Lonely

Nursing diagnosis_____

Verbal_____

Nonverbal_____

Out of control

Nursing diagnosis_____

Verbal_____

Nonverbal_____

For each of the following roles, pretend the role has been disrupted due to a health problem. Write a possible psycho-social-cultural nursing diagnosis and a sentence about a situation in which this diagnosis would be appropriate. As a critical thinking exercise, use a different diagnosis for each role alteration. There are a number of different diagnoses that could be appropriate depending on the situation:

Worker:

Nursing diagnosis_____

Rationale_____

Student:

Nursing diagnosis_____

Rationale_____

Parent:

Nursing diagnosis_____

Rationale_____

Husband/Wife:

Nursing diagnosis_____

Rationale_____

Lover:

Nursing diagnosis_____

Rationale_____

Friend:

Nursing diagnosis_____

Rationale_____

Son/Daughter:

Nursing diagnosis_____

Rationale_____

Sister/brother:

Nursing diagnosis_____

Rationale_____

Grandparent:

Nursing diagnosis_____

Rationale_____

For each of the following psychosocial problems involving an interaction with the health-care provider, give a psychosocial nursing diagnosis. Write a sentence about why this diagnosis would be appropriate. As this is a critical-thinking exercise, use a different diagnosis for each situation.

The patient signs himself out of the hospital against medical advice.

Nursing diagnosis_____

Rationale_____

The family cannot decide whether to permit the patient to have a feeding tube.

Nursing diagnosis_____

Rationale_____

The family cannot handle all the care required for the ventilator-dependent child at home.

Nursing diagnosis_____

Rationale_____

The cardiac patient states she has no time to do her exercise prescription.

Nursing diagnosis_____

Rationale_____

For each of the following situations, which involve changes in body image or self-esteem, give a possible psychosocial nursing diagnosis, and write a sentence about why this diagnosis would be appropriate. Use a different diagnosis for each alteration.

The patient refuses to look at the appendectomy scar.

Nursing diagnosis_____

Rationale_____

The patient with a heart attack states, "I'm just no good anymore, I'll never be able to go back to my old job."

Nursing diagnosis_____

Rationale_____

"I'm so ashamed of the way I look without my hair since the chemotherapy."

Nursing diagnosis_____

Rationale_____

"I haven't been outside this apartment for six months because I'm a cripple and I don't want anyone to see me."

Nursing diagnosis_____

Rationale_____

For each of the following examples of cultural nursing care problems, give a possible nursing diagnosis, and write a sentence about why this diagnosis would be appropriate. Use a different diagnosis for each alteration.

The patient says she cannot understand how God could have let this happen to her.

Nursing diagnosis_____

Rationale_____

An East Indian woman arrives by ambulance to Labor and Delivery and screams with each contraction. She does not understand English, and there is no interpreter available. Her husband is on the way to the hospital.

Nursing diagnosis_____

Rationale_____

The Jehovah's Witness with a hemoglobin level of 5 is actively bleeding and refuses blood.

Nursing diagnosis_____

Rationale_____

5. Practice therapeutic communication techniques by completing the exercise below.

Following are gender communication examples. Specify whether they are typical male or female patterns of communication. Write why you think so and your response.

The physician comes into the room, says hello, and asks, "What's going on with Mrs. G?"

_____

The nurse says to the patient, "It's time to get up to sit in a chair, don't you think so?"

_____

The patient says to the nurse, "I'm sorry to be such a bother to you."

_____

Mini Cultural Assessment: Please assess yourself, then exchange views with others from similar and different cultural backgrounds.

1. What people from cultural/ethnic groups have you become friends with?
2. In what country were you born?
3. In what countries did your ancestors originate on your mother's and father's sides of your family?
4. How closely do you associate with your parents and grandparents?
5. Whom do you consider your family? Relatives, friends, pets?
6. How important is your family to you?
7. In your family, who takes care of infants and children? Who spends the most time taking care of them?
8. In your family, who takes care of the sick or elderly? Who spends the most time taking care of them?
9. Describe your thoughts and feelings about marriage.
10. Describe your thoughts and feelings about childbearing.
11. Should a mother nurse her baby in public or private? Should babies be breastfed?
12. The environment refers to the planet Earth and the communities in which people live. Should we preserve or use the resources? Should we recycle?
13. What is the meaning of life? Explain. Why are people put on Earth?
14. What do you think about death? What happens when you die?
15. How important is punctuality to you? Should people be on time?
16. What do you think about the past? Is what happened in the past relevant to the present?
17. What do you think about the present? Should we live "for the moment"?
18. What do you think about the future? What should the future bring?
19. Is money and having status important?
20. Who does the cooking, cleaning, yard work, care maintenance in your family?
21. How are decisions made in your family? Are steps of problem solving followed in your family? Explain how decisions are made in your family.
22. What place do elderly relatives have in your life?
23. Is the sex of a baby important? Are girls and boys treated differently as they grow?
24. What rules govern sexual activity for a man? For a woman?

● Figure 6.6   Mini cultural assessment. (Adapted from Schuster, P: Communication: The Key to the Therapeutic Relationship. FA Davis, Philadelphia, 2000, with permission.)

REFERENCES

1. Erickson, EH: The Life Cycle Completed. Norton, New York, 1998.
2. Satir, V: New Peoplemaking. Science and Behavior Books, Palo Alto, California, 1988 (seminal book).
3. Purnell, LD, and Paulanda, BJ: Transcultural Health Care: A Culturally Competent Approach, ed 2. FA Davis, Philadelphia, 2003.
4. Tannen, D: You Just Don't Understand: Women and Men in Conversation. Ballantine, New York, 1990 (seminal book).
5. Schuster, PM: Communication: The Key to the Therapeutic Relationship. FA Davis, Philadelphia, 2000.

7

CONCEPT CARE MAPS AS THE BASIS OF DOCUMENTATION AND PHONE CONVERSATIONS WITH PHYSICIANS

OBJECTIVES

1. List purposes of documentation.

2. Describe the relationships between the American Nurses Association standards of care, American Nurses Association documentation standards, and concept care maps.

3. Specify the basic content of nursing care documentation.

4. Compare documentation formats for standardized forms and narrative progress notes.

5. Identify basic criteria that guide documentation.

6. Use the concept care map to identify content for documentation.

7. Describe the purpose of HIPAA and documentation.

8. Use the concept care map to develop the SBAR to communicate with physicians and document the conversation.

The purposes of this chapter are to provide basic information about the process of basic documentation and to explain the use of concept care maps as guides for documentation. Documentation, also known as charting, is the legal record of written communication of all patient care activities from each health-care provider involved in the patient's care. It is crucial that nursing students know how to document accurately and efficiently. This chapter provides a very basic guide to documentation, and nursing students will be given very specific documentation guidelines during clinical rotations to differing health-care facilities and also as they change units within the same health-care facility.

Nurses are legally accountable for following nursing standards of care, and documentation is the written evidence that standards of care were followed. This is also the situation for all other health-care providers involved in patient care. All providers must follow standards of care for their own professional disciplines and provide written evidence that standards were met. Should there be a malpractice claim, charts will be subpoenaed in court, and this legal record may be used as evidence of the health-care services provided and the patient's responses to those services.

Administrators of health-care agencies use patient records to conduct quality assurance audits to monitor the effectiveness and efficiency of all services. Written documentation is needed to ensure quality of patient care by supplying evidence to administrators that health-care providers are doing their jobs. Health administrators are interested in maintaining accreditation by the Joint Commission on Accreditation of Healthcare Organizations (JCAHO). Administrators enforce the strict standards of documentation dictated by the JCAHO. Administrators are also focused on collecting money from insurance companies, managed care organizations, Medicare, and Medicaid for services provided. The amount of reimbursement is based on documentation. Failure to document provided services correctly results in lack of appropriate reimbursement.

Everything that was written on the concept care map is documented somewhere in the patient records. Information must be documented concerning all medical and nursing diagnoses that have been identified in the concept care map, through use of flow sheets, progress notes, or care plans. Steps 1, 2, and 3 of concept care mapping, involving development of the diagram, will be used as the basis for documentation of assessment data. Step 4, involving outcomes and interventions, will be used to guide documentation of implementation of nursing interventions to attain outcomes. Step 5, notes on the evaluation of patient responses to nursing interventions, will be used to guide documentation of patient responses and progress toward outcome objectives. Documentation is a challenge for every health-care provider. Formats for documentation and the exact procedures for documentation are in a constant state of flux. However, the concept care maps are very useful tools to help you focus on the basic content of what must be documented.

What to Document

The primary objective is to provide evidence that practice standards have been upheld. It is also a form of communication with other health-care providers and a way to ensure the best, most seamless health-care provision possible. Assessments, diagnoses, outcomes, interventions, and patient responses must be documented for each encounter with a patient.

Nurses must understand the relationships among documentation standards, care standards of the American Nurses Association (ANA),[1] and concept care maps. Linkages between care standards, documentation standards, and concept map care plans are shown in Figure 7.1. Concept care maps facilitate documentation because they are cohesive, written, individualized summaries of patient care based on standards of practice.

In summary, documentation standards require that patient care assessment data be documented in retrievable form. Nursing and medical diagnoses must be included and must be documented in a manner that facilitates determination of expected patient outcomes. Patient outcomes need to be documented as measurable goals. There must be a written plan of care with specified interventions and active patient participation in development of the care plan. All interventions that are implemented must be documented. All reassessments and revisions in

---

ANA Standards of Care Relevant to Documentation

Standard 1. **Assessment:** The nurse collects patient health data.
Documentation: Data are documented in a retrievable form.
Concept map: Assessment data are collected using the patient profile assessment guidelines. Priority assessment data are summarized on the diagram under nursing and medical diagnoses.

Standard 2. **Diagnoses:** The nurse analyzes the assessment data in determining diagnoses.
Documentation: Diagnoses are documented in a manner that facilitates the determination of expected outcomes and plan of care.
Concept map: Nursing diagnoses formulated using Steps 1 to 3 of the concept map care planning process are numbered on the diagram to correspond with the outcomes in Step 4.

Standard 3. **Outcome identification:** The nurse identifies expected goals and outcomes individualized to the patient.
Documentation: Outcomes are documented as measurable goals.
Concept map: Individualized outcomes are specified in Step 4.

Standards 4 and 5. **Planning:** The nurse develops a plan of care that prescribes interventions to attain expected outcomes with active patient participation in health promotions, maintenance, and restoration.
Documentation: The plan is documented.
Concept map plan: Interventions and outcomes are listed in Step 4.

Standard 6. **Implementation:** The nurse implements the interventions identified in the plan of care to maximize health capabilities.
Documentation: Interventions are documented.
Concept map: Interventions are listed in Step 4 under goals/objectives, and as interventions are completed, they are checked off as done.

Standards 7 and 8. **Evaluation:** The nurse and patient evaluate the patient's progress toward attainment of outcomes, with reordering of priorities, new goal setting, and revision of the nursing care plan as needed to attain health goals.
Documentation: Reassessments and revisions in diagnoses, outcomes, and the plan of care are documented. The patient's responses to interventions are documented.
Concept map: Step 5 of the concept map involves the patient's responses to interventions. All revisions written on the concept map are delineated by using ink that is a different color from the initial care plan.

Based on Nursing's Social Policy Statement, ed 2. American Nurses Association, nursesbooks.org, Washington, D.C., 2003.

● Figure 7.1 ANA standards of care relevant to documentation.

diagnoses, outcomes, and the plan of care are documented. Documentation includes patient's responses to interventions.

Where to Document

Everything on the care map needs to be documented somewhere. It is initially overwhelming to think that everything has to be recorded in medical records. However, not everything has to be personally typed into a computer or written down by your own hand, word by word. Healthcare agencies provide nurses with standardized forms to accomplish the daunting task of documentation (Fig. 7.2). In addition, succinct written narrative comments are recorded on progress note forms (Fig. 7.3).

Forum
HEALTH

MEDICAL/SURGICAL FLOW SHEET   DATE _____

V S	**TIME**																			
I I	Temperature																			
T G	Pulse																			
A N	Respirations																			
L S	Blood Pressure																			
	MENTAL STATUS																			
	PAIN																			
A	**RESP STATUS** Breath Sounds																			
	Type																			
S	**G.I. STATUS** Bowel Sounds																			
S	Abdomen																			
E	**PERIPHERAL**	R L	R L	R L	R L	R L	R L	R L	R L	R L	R L	R L	R L	R L	R L	R L	R L
S	**VASCULAR** Radial																			
S	**STATUS** Dorsalis Pedis																			
M	**INTEGUMENTARY** Color/Temp																			
	STATUS Wound/Lesion																			
E	DUP SCORE **Every Monday**																			
	IV SITE_____ /RATE																			
N	IV SITE_____ /RATE																			
	MOBILITY																			
T	FALLS SCORE **Every Monday**																			
	R.N. INITIALS																			
	ACTIVITY/SAFETY Bedrest																			
	Turn																			
I	ROM																			
	Leg Exercises																			
N	Chair																			
	Ambulation																			
T	Bathroom																			
	BSC																			
E	Bedpan/Urinal																			
	Siderails/Call Light																			
R	HOB ↑																			
V	**HYGIENE** Bath/Shower																			
	HS/Back Care																			
E	Mouth Care																			
	Cath Care																			
N	**DIET** Consumed																			
	Method																			
T	NPO/HS Snack																			
	TUBE FEEDING Rate																			
I	Residual Check																			
	Tube Placement Check																			
O	**TREATMENTS** DB and Cough																			
	TED Hose/Binder																			
N	**RESTRAINT CHECK** Level_____																			
S																				

CODES

* Needs further explanation

Pulse
AP - Apical pulse
R - Regular
I - Irregular*

Temperature
AX - Axillary temp
R - Rectal temp
T - Tympanic

Mental Status
A = Alert/0x3
S = Sleeping
O = Other*

Pain
0 = None
Scale 1-10*

Bowel Sounds
N = Normal
0 = Absent*
↑ = Increased*
↓ = Decreased*

Pulses
0 = Absent*
1+ = Weak*
        Thready
2+ = Decreased*
3+ = Normal
4+ = Bounding

Mobility
N = Normal
I = Impaired*

Activity/Hygiene/Turn/Pos
L = Left Side   S = Self
R = Right Side   A = Assist
B = Back   C = Complete
P = Prone

Consumed
G = Good 80-100%   **Method**
F = Fair 60-80%   S = Self
P = Poor 60%   A = Assist
                     F = Feed

Resp. Type
N = Normal
S = Shallow*
D = Deep
L = Labored

Breath Sounds
C = Clear
Rh = Rhonchi*
Ra = Rales*
Wz = Wheeze*

Abdomen
S = Soft
D = Distended*
F = Firm*

Skin Temp
W = Warm/Dry
C = Cool
D = Diaphoretic*

Skin Color
N = Normal
C = Cyanotic*
J = Jaundiced*
O = Other*

Wound/Lesion
N = None
O = Other*

Tube Feeding
C = Continuous
B = Bolus
I = Intermittent

Level I Restraint Check includes:
• Visual observation
• Restraint placement
• *Other

Level II & III Restraint Check includes:
• Visual observation
• Restraint placement
• Color/Temperature Check
• Restraint Release for 10 min. q 2 h
• Activity/ROM
• The offer for toileting and norishment/fluids
• Mental Status
• *Other

Initials	Signature	Shift R.N.

7301005 Rev. 12/97

Flow sheet column labels:

TIME — VITAL SIGNS: Temperature, Pulse, Respirations, Blood Pressure

MENTAL STATUS / PAIN

ASSESSMENT:
RESP STATUS — Breath Sounds, Type
GI STATUS — Bowel Sounds, Abdomen
PERIPHERAL VASCULAR STATUS — Radial (R L), Dorsalis Pedis (R L)
INTEGUMENTARY STATUS — Color/Temp, Wound/Lesion
DUP SCORE [Every Monday]
IV SITE ____ /RATE
IV SITE ____ /RATE
MOBILITY
FALLS SCORE [Every Monday]
R.N. INITIALS

INTERVENTIONS:
ACTIVITY/SAFETY — Bedrest, Turn, ROM, Leg Exercises, Chair, Ambulation, Bathroom, BSC, Bedpan/Urinal, Siderails/Call Light, HOB ↑
HYGIENE — Bath/Shower, HS/Back Care, Mouth Care, Cath Care
DIET — Consumed, Method, NPO/HS Snack
TUBE FEEDING — Rate, Residual Check, Tube Placement Check
TREATMENTS — DB and Cough, TED Hose/Binder
RESTRAINT CHECK

● Figure 7.2   Sample flow sheet (Forum Health, Youngstown, Ohio, with permission).

Date/Time HOUR	P.R.N. and Stat Medication	NOTES
9-8-08		
0800		Reports pain in surgical incision area "5" on "10"
		point scale, requests pain medication. N Direnzo, 1/SU, SN —
0810		Given 2 vicodin for pain w/ instruction on use
		of visual imagery exercises & slow deep breathing.
		N Direnzo, 1/SU, SN —
0900		Reports pain is now "2". N Direnzo, 1/SU, SN —

Jorum HEALTH

NURSES NOTES
USE "MIDNIGHT LINE" FOR DATING THE NEW DAY

Addressograph

7301811

● Figure 7.3   Sample nurse's notes.

Standardized Paper or Computerized Forms

You must become familiar with the standardized and computerized forms that provide the basis of documentation in each health-care facility. Standardized forms increase consistency and the completeness of information gathered and decrease time spent on documentation. Typical formats of standardized forms include checklists and fill-ins with space for a few words. Blank sections are provided for expanding on and clarifying information to allow individualization of care. As you gain clinical experience at different health-care agencies, you will note many similarities in the contents of standardized forms. Although contents are similar, the layout varies. You will also be expected to record documentation information on the flow sheets and progress notes used by the health-care facility.

Documentation Standards for Assessment and Reassessment

There are many standardized forms for the assessment and reassessment of patients to accomplish documentation Standard 1 that all data are documented in a retrievable form. There are standardized forms used for the continual assessment and evaluation of the care of patients, which include history and physical admission assessments and specialized, customized key assessments that occur on an ongoing basis. When assessments are ongoing, they are considered reassessments. You can also think of the reassessments as data for continued evaluation of patient responses to nursing interventions. The terminology gets a bit confusing, but after an initial assessment, nurses continue to assess in order to evaluate responses to nursing interventions.

As patients enter the inpatient or outpatient health-care system for the first time, there will be a comprehensive history and physical done on admission, with subsequent key reassessments customized to the health problems. For example, for a patient with hypertension, the focus of key subsequent assessments will be on the cardiovascular system. Each area of care, such as medical units, surgical units, outpatient clinics, pediatric clinics, and geriatric units, will

conduct a complete history and physical and then focus on follow-up reassessments by collecting data specific to the type of patient care provided by the facility.

Assessments and Standardized Flow Sheets

Flow sheets are a special type of standardized form used for frequent assessments or reassessments. Nurses always start with a baseline assessment. Subsequent assessments of the same parameter are considered reassessments, but may also be considered evaluation data. As examples, assessment of neurological checks and vital signs are tracked with flow sheets. Flow sheets have formats that allow key data to be seen either in columns or rows and tracked over time. Flow sheets allow easy comparisons to determine trends in assessment data over time. A sample flow sheet is shown in Figure 7.2.

Linking Concept Care Maps to Documentation of Assessment and Reassessments

The concept care map is useful to guide ongoing assessments, reassessments, and evaluations on agency standardized documentation forms. Step 5 of the concept care map contains information you have written on patient responses, which are reassessments of what was initially assessed using the patient profile database. Make sure you know where to document assessment and reassessment information on the agency's standardized forms.

Documentation Standards for Nursing Diagnoses and Care Plans

The purpose of developing care plans is to communicate diagnoses, goals, and outcomes of care; coordinate patient care; and ensure continuity of care.

In 1992 JCAHO accreditation standards changed requirements from an individualized plan of nursing care for each patient to recording data about assessments, diagnoses, or patient needs, nursing interventions, and patient outcomes (Standard NC 1.3.5) on the patient medical records.[2] Many health-care agencies have developed standardized care plans for patients with specific diagnoses in order to decrease paperwork and to meet the ANA and JCAHO standards for practice and documentation. Historically, health-care agencies and nursing schools used a standardized care plan format that has four columns for nursing diagnoses: patient/family outcomes, nursing interventions, rationales for interventions, and evaluation of outcomes (Fig. 7.4).

Nurses need only check, date, and sign appropriate columns in the plan to save time writing about routine outcomes, interventions, rationales, and evaluation of outcomes. Space is usually provided on the standardized forms for individualized outcomes and interventions. A sample standardized care plan from a hospital is shown in Figure 7.5.

Standardized care plans are useful for nurses and student nurses who are inexperienced in caring for patients with particular diagnoses because expected outcomes and interventions are clearly evident. In each agency you are assigned for clinical experiences, you need to locate and study standardized care plans that may be computer-

ized or preprinted. If care plans are not available, there are numerous up-to-date standardized nursing care plan texts available as well as medical-surgical texts containing standardized plans of care to guide you in developing the individualized concept care maps. Experienced nurses have the outcomes, interventions, and rationales ingrained from practice and thus have little use for standardized plans of care. There are still numerous complaints from nurses that standardized nursing care plans are just extra paperwork to check, date, and sign.

The current trend in care planning is for agencies to develop and use the standardized interdisciplinary care plans called critical or clinical pathways. These are based on outcomes for specific patient problems such as knee replacements. They have been developed by teams of health-care providers involved in the care of a specific patient population. As with other standardized care plans, nurses need only

Nursing Diagnoses	Patient/Family Outcomes	Nursing Intervention	Rationale for Interventions	Evaluation of Outcomes
# _____ Diagnosis _____ Definition _____ _____ _____ Defining characteristics of your specific patient ____ _____ _____ _____ Related factors of your specific patient _____ _____ _____ _____ General goal: _____ _____ _____ _____	Outcome statement with measurable, time limited, specific, individual objectives. The patient will: 1a _____ _____ _____on the day of care. The patient will: 1b _____ _____ _____on the day of care. The patient will: 1c _____ _____ _____on the day of care. The patient will: 1d _____ _____ _____on the day of care. The patient will: 1e _____ _____ _____on the day of care.	The nurse will: 1a _____ _____ _____ 1b _____ _____ _____ 1c _____ _____ _____ 1d _____ _____ _____ 1e _____ _____ _____	1a _____ _____ _____ 1b _____ _____ _____ 1c _____ _____ _____ 1d _____ _____ _____ 1e _____ _____ _____	1a _____ _____ _____ 1b _____ _____ _____ 1c _____ _____ _____ 1d _____ _____ _____ 1e _____ _____ _____

● Figure 7.4 Sample column patient care plan.

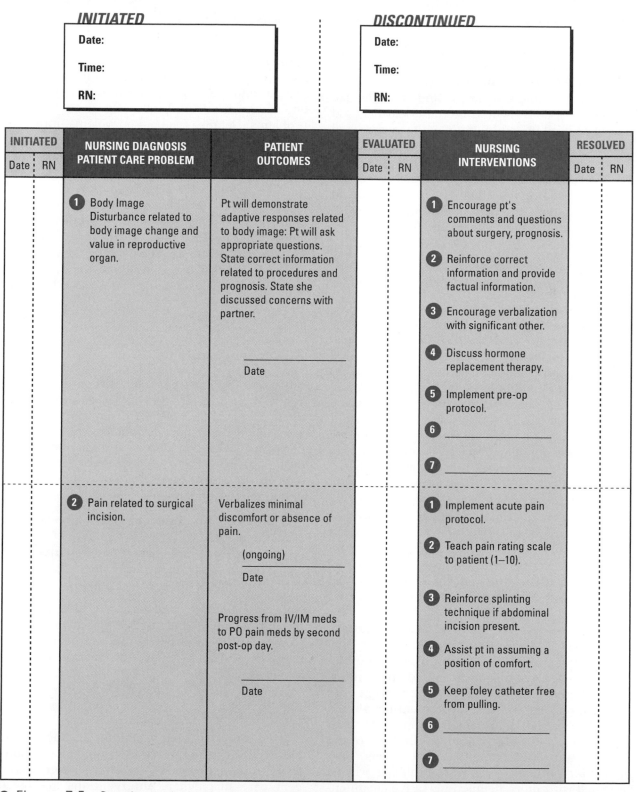

INITIATED

Date:

Time:

RN:

DISCONTINUED

Date:

Time:

RN:

INITIATED		NURSING DIAGNOSIS PATIENT CARE PROBLEM	PATIENT OUTCOMES	EVALUATED		NURSING INTERVENTIONS	RESOLVED	
Date	RN			Date	RN		Date	RN
		1 Body Image Disturbance related to body image change and value in reproductive organ.	Pt will demonstrate adaptive responses related to body image: Pt will ask appropriate questions. State correct information related to procedures and prognosis. State she discussed concerns with partner. _____ Date			**1** Encourage pt's comments and questions about surgery, prognosis. **2** Reinforce correct information and provide factual information. **3** Encourage verbalization with significant other. **4** Discuss hormone replacement therapy. **5** Implement pre-op protocol. **6** _____ **7** _____		
		2 Pain related to surgical incision.	Verbalizes minimal discomfort or absence of pain. (ongoing) _____ Date Progress from IV/IM meds to PO pain meds by second post-op day. _____ Date			**1** Implement acute pain protocol. **2** Teach pain rating scale to patient (1–10). **3** Reinforce splinting technique if abdominal incision present. **4** Assist pt in assuming a position of comfort. **5** Keep foley catheter free from pulling. **6** _____ **7** _____		

● Figure 7.5   Sample standardized care plan. (Modified from Forum Health, Youngstown, Ohio, with permission.)

check, date, and sign appropriate columns of the care plan.

Linking Concept Care Maps to Documentation on Standardized Column Care Plans

Concept care maps organize and individualize nursing care delivery and increase learning and should be used in combination with standardized column care plans. At the clinical agencies, use the concept care map to individualize the standardized care plans. If there are diagnoses on the diagram that are not included in standardized plans, add them to the standardized plan with appropriate outcomes and interventions.

Documentation Standards for Implementation of Nursing Interventions

Standard treatments, medications, and intravenous (IV) fluids are documented on flow sheets. Examples of standard treatments in hospital settings include bath, back care, and oral care. Space is provided on standardized forms for additional treatments to individualize the plan of care. Nursing interventions, such as administering medications and IV fluids, are very important nursing activities, and they must be documented carefully using medication and IV administration flow sheets. For example, the antibiotic administered over 3 days is tracked from time to time and day to day across a row of a medication flow sheet. All prn (as needed) medications will be documented on the flow sheets and also expanded upon in the narrative notes. Documentation of treatments, medications, and IV therapy is done by listing the dates and times in the appropriate spaces on the flow sheets.

Linking Concept Care Maps to Documentation on Standard Intervention Flow Sheets

Interventions are listed on the front of the diagram under each diagnosis. In addition, interventions are listed in step 4 of the concept care map. All ongoing treatment interventions should be listed on the treatment flow sheet. Medications and IVs are highlighted on the front of the diagram and documented on flow sheets. Specific interventions to alleviate problems will be included with more detailed narrative documentation of specific problems. A sample flow sheet with assessments and interventions is shown in Figure 7.2.

Documentation of Specific Problems: Easy as PIE

Standardized forms for assessment, reassessments/evaluations, and interventions save a lot of time and organize information. There is not enough room on the forms to go into detail for problems. Details of specific problems, interventions, and patient responses are expanded upon using progress notes (also called narrative notes), shown in Figure 7.3.

The content of documentation of specific problems can be determined easily using the concept care map diagram of problems as a guide. Each nursing diagnosis must be described in the progress notes. For each nursing diagnosis, documentation can be done in three steps that are as easy as PIE: first, describe the Problem; then, write Interventions; finally, Evaluate patient responses.[3]

Progress Note P

First, list the nursing diagnosis, and then describe the problem by writing abnormal assessment data that support the diagnosis. Abnormal assessment/reassessment data are located on the diagram of the concept care map under each diagnosis. In addition, assessment/reassessment data are located in step 5, patient responses/evaluation of the concept care map. For example:

> 2/11/07 8 a.m. Problem: pain (surgical incision)
> *Reports pain in surgical incision area 5 on 10-point scale; requests medication. N. DiRenzo, YSU, SN*

Note that the date and time are first, followed by the diagnosis and assessment data. In this example, the information is subjective, because it indicates what the patient reported about pain.

Progress Note I

Second, describe what was done to alleviate the problem. Write all interventions and instructions given to the patient. "I" corresponds to the concept care map where interventions are listed under the diagnoses. In addition, interventions are listed in step 4 of the concept care map. For example:

*8:10 a.m. Given 2 Vicodin (hydrocodone/
acetaminophen) for pain w/instruction
on visual imagery exercises. N. DiRenzo,
YSU, SN*

Progress Note E

Third, describe the patient response to the nursing interventions that were done. This entails reassessment and evaluation of the initial assessment data. Evaluation of patient responses to nursing interventions is listed in step 5 of the concept care map. For example:

*9:00 a.m. Reports pain is now 2. N.
DiRenzo, YSU, SN*

In the actual progress notes (with explanations deleted), the entry would look like this:

*2/11/07 8 a.m. Problem: pain (surgical
incision)
Reports pain in surgical incision area 5 on
10-point scale; requests medication. N.
DiRenzo, YSU, SN
8:10 a.m. Given 2 Vicodin (hydrocodone/
acetaminophen) for pain w/instruction
on visual imagery exercises. N. DiRenzo,
YSU, SN
9:00 a.m. Reports pain is now 2. N.
DiRenzo, YSU, SN*

The preceding example shows the basics of the PIE documentation, but sometimes problems do not resolve as easily. In the next example, the initial interventions do not work to alleviate the problem, so more interventions are performed, and patient responses are again evaluated (reassessed).

*2/11/07 8 a.m. problem: Constipation
(postoperative decreased GI motility)
Reports unable to have BM in 3 days and
abdominal discomfort is 3 on a 10-point
scale, belching and passing flatus +
bowel sounds 4 quadrants. N. DiRenzo,
YSU, SN
8:10 a.m. Given 30 cc MOM (magnesium
hydroxide), instructed to drink more
water, and given warm tea to drink. N.
DiRenzo, YSU, SN
10 a.m. Bowel assessment unchanged
from 8 a.m. N. DiRenzo, YSU, SN*

Unfortunately, constipation is not alleviated by using milk of magnesia or by drinking water and

tea; additional interventions are therefore needed. It frequently occurs that you will need to continue to work on a problem throughout the day. The nurse has reassessed/evaluated the outcome and now has to intervene and document additional "I" interventions. There is an ongoing problem, so the evaluation becomes a reassessment and leads directly to the need for additional interventions. This is followed by reassessment/evaluation in the following example:

Write Another Progress Note I

What was done next?

*10:10 a.m. Given Fleet enema. N. DiRenzo,
YSU, SN*

Write Another Progress Note E

Patient response now?

*10:15 a.m. Large brown formed BM per
bedside commode. Patient reports feeling
better, discomfort 0. N. DiRenzo, YSU, SN*

This popular documentation system of using standardized forms with progress notes to give details on problems has been termed "documentation by exception" and a "problem-oriented approach."[4] Checklists and fill-ins are useful for quickly recording assessments, interventions, and evaluations. Problems identified are then expanded in the progress notes. There is no need to write details about assessments/evaluations that are within normal limits. It is only necessary to write about exceptions to the norm.

It is very important to be able to provide an in-depth description of the problems with interventions and evaluation of patient responses to nursing interventions.

Mnemonics (memory aids) in addition to PIE include DAR and SOAPIER. The information contained in the entries is the same. DAR denotes:

- Problem assessment *Data*
- Nursing *Actions*
- Evaluation of *Responses*

SOAPIER denotes:

- Subjective and Objective Data
- Assessments
- Plan
- Interventions
- Evaluations
- Revisions

How to Document: Basic Criteria

Good documentation is concise, accurate, complete, legible, timely, and logically organized. These criteria must be applied each time the nurse makes an entry on a chart.[5]

Accuracy of Patient Name, Dates, and Times

Each time something is recorded, the date and time must be included. Check to ensure that the patient's name is on all sheets on which you are recording information. For the same problems, be sure that the dates and times on the flow sheets match the dates and times in the progress notes.

A 24-hour clock, often referred to as military time, is used in most health-care facilities to clearly distinguish a.m. from p.m. hours (Table 7.1).

Accuracy of Entries

Always use objective and measurable terms about the patient's behaviors and speech. Objective data include something you heard, saw, felt, or smelled, termed empirical sensory data. This information is strictly factual; it is not appropriate to write opinions, biased statements, or speculations. For example, if you label the patient "a complainer," you may miss important assessment information. Instead, write a quote about what the patient stated. Write only what you see, and let the reader draw any conclusions.

Table 7.1 **24-Hour Clock**	
1 p.m. = 1300	1 a.m. = 0100
2 p.m. = 1400	2 a.m. = 0200
3 p.m. = 1500	3 a.m. = 0300
4 p.m. = 1600	4 a.m. = 0400
5 p.m. = 1700	5 a.m. = 0500
6 p.m. = 1800	6 a.m. = 0600
7 p.m. = 1900	7 a.m. = 0700
8 p.m. = 2000	8 a.m. = 0800
9 p.m. = 2100	9 a.m. = 0900
10 p.m. = 2200	10 a.m. = 1000
11 p.m. = 2300	11 a.m. = 1100
12 midnight = 2400	12 noon = 1200

Remember, patients have the right to read their charts at any time.

Legibility

All entries must be legible and in black ink. Write neatly, spell correctly, and write on the lines provided. Ink is used because it cannot be erased and can be photocopied. Illegible writing can lead to life-threatening situations, such as medication errors. Always question and clarify illegible writing to avoid patient-care errors. Illegible medication and treatment orders are especially dangerous. In addition, start entries with a capital letter and end with a period.

Signatures

Always sign the document carefully, using the first letter of your first name, your last name, and title. Traditionally, SN has been the abbreviation for student nurse, LPN for licensed practical nurse, and RN for registered nurse. Because many nursing schools may share the same facility, you will be required to write the abbreviation of your school affiliation along with the title SN; for example N. DiRenzo, YSU, SN.

Never sign anyone else's entry. You are accountable for whatever you sign. The only exception is if a caregiver has left the health-care agency for the day and calls in with information she forgot to document. Then the conversation must be documented in the progress notes, and corrections must be made on the records.

Correcting Mistakes

When you make a mistake, draw a single line through the words, write *error* above the words, and sign your name or initials. Then make the correct entry. Always correct documentation errors promptly in order to avoid patient care errors. Never erase entries; never use correction fluid, or never scribble errors. It should not look like data were hidden or tampered with in any way.

Logical Organization of Information

To ensure correct sequencing of events, document on the standardized forms and progress notes as you go throughout the day. Do not wait until the end of the day to record what happened with patients. It is much easier to accurately remember the sequence of events if you record them shortly after occurrence. Also, do not document in advance. Other health-care providers are dependent on information you document to implement their plans of care, and there is potential for patient care errors when documentation is not timely or accurate.

Always chart consecutively, line by line, in the progress notes. Never leave blank spaces in progress notes. If you leave blanks, another health-care provider can add incorrect information to the spaces. If space is left after you sign and date an entry, draw a line out to the right margin of the line.

Writing a Late Entry

Sometimes the nurse may forget to write some information that needs to be included. Start the late entry with the current month, date and time, and then write "Addendum to nurse's note of (month)/(date)/(time)." Never try to squeeze in additional notes near previously written notes. Always make addenda when you forget to enter information. A well-known rule of thumb to guide documentation is: "If you didn't chart it, it wasn't done."

Completeness

All standardized forms must be filled in completely, with spaces filled in with "not applicable" (NA) if it does not apply to the patient. For example, menstrual cycle information is not applicable for male patients, and the blank is filled in with NA.

Overgeneralizations can also be problematic. Specific information is needed. For example, what does "not having a good day" mean exactly? Overgeneralizations waste space, lack objectivity, and are incomplete.

Omitted Interventions

Sometimes interventions are purposely omitted because of the patient's condition or unavailability of the patient. For example, the patient has a daily laxative scheduled as a routine medication, but the patient now reports loose stools, so the nurse does not give the medication. The reason the drug is not given must be included in a progress note, and an order must be obtained from the physician to discontinue the drug. Sometimes the patient may be off the unit when drugs are supposed to be given, so drugs are not given on time; a note must be made why the drugs were not given at the specified time. Omissions without explanations are considered errors because, legally, you must do all you are supposed to do or give an explanation why something is not done and then notify the appropriate members of the health-care team.

Conciseness

Charting entries must be brief, using incomplete sentences. Eliminate all words that do not change the intended meaning of the entry, including articles such as "a" and "the," and also the subject of the sentence. Use standard abbreviations for conciseness but only those that are approved by the health-care agency. You can write patient or family comments, but you must put quotes around the actual words the patient spoke. The sample PIE documentations given above are examples of concise entries. Note that neither the patient's name nor the word "patient" was charted because all entries are about the patient. Also, it is a waste of time and space to repeat in a narrative statement in the progress notes what was covered sufficiently on standardized forms.

Confidentiality

Patient privacy has always been an important part of nursing responsibilities. Patient information must be confidential, and documentation systems must be secure. The Health Insurance Portability and Accountability Act (HIPAA) was established to protect patient privacy for written and electronic documentation. This 1996 legislation maintains the security of health information about patients. Prior to this act, many patients did not know that their medical records could be released to other parties such as insurance companies, employers, or researchers without permission from patients. Nurses have always been patient advocates for privacy, and now there are specific laws to protect privacy.[6]

Documentation of Communication With Physicians and Other Health-Care Providers

JCAHO has reported that communication errors are the root cause of 70% of sentinel events.[7] Sentinel events are defined as those having serious physical or psychological injury or death. Nurses must learn to give concise and informative verbal reports to physicians. Nurses are sometimes afraid to call certain physicians because they fear they will be reprimanded for being ill-timed or uninformative. Physicians complain about nurses calling inappropriately, and nurses complain about rude disruptive behavior from physicians during telephone conversations. Nurses may delay care because they are afraid to call physicians. The style of nursing communication is often broad and narrative, when physicians are interested in a brief succinct report.

The communication problem has resulted in the development of the SBAR shared communication model for nurses to use when giving telephone reports to physicians.[8] SBAR stands for *S*ituation-*B*ackground-*A*ssessment-*R*ecommendation. The concept care map contains all the information needed for the SBAR tool. The Institute for Healthcare Improvement provides guidelines for communicating with physicians using the SBAR process, shown in Table 7.2. This table provides a step-by-step guide for what to say as you give a patient report to a physician. The template for the SBAR report to a physician about a critical situation is shown in Figure 7.6.

Table 7.2 Guidelines for Communication With Physicians Using the SBAR Process

1. Use the following modalities according to physician preference, if known. Wait no longer than 5 minutes between attempts.
   - Direct page (if known)
   - Physician's call service
   - During weekdays, the physician's office directly
   - On weekends and after hours during the week, physician's home phone
   - Cell phone
   Before assuming that the physician you are attempting to reach is not responding, utilize all modalities. For emergent situations, use appropriate resident service as needed to ensure safe patient care.
2. Prior to calling the physician, follow these steps:
   - Have I seen and assessed the patient myself before calling?
   - Has the situation been discussed with resource nurse or preceptor?
   - Review the chart for appropriate physician to call.
   - Know the admitting diagnosis and date of admission.
   - Have I read the most recent MD progress notes and notes from the nurse who worked the shift ahead of me?
   - Have available the following when speaking with the physician: patient's chart; list of current medications, allergies, IV fluids, and laboratory test results (provide the date and time test was done and results of previous tests for comparison); most recent vital signs; code status
3. When calling the physician, follow the SBAR process:
   *S*ituation: What is the situation you are calling about?
   - Identify self, unit, patient, room number
   - Briefly state the problem, when it happened or started, and how severe
   *B*ackground: Pertinent background information related to the situation could include the following:
   - The admitting diagnosis and date of admission
   - List of current medications, allergies, IV fluids, and laboratory test results (provide the date and time test was done and results of previous tests for comparison)
   - Most recent vital signs
   - Other clinical information
   - Code status
   *A*ssessment: What is the nurse's assessment of the situation?
   *R*ecommendation: What is the nurse's recommendation or what does he/she want?
   Examples:
   - Notification that patient has been admitted
   - Patient needs to be seen now
   - Order change
4. Document the change in the patient's condition and physician notification.

SBAR report to physician about a critical situation

S	**Situation**
	I am calling about \<patient's name and location>
	The patient's code status is \<code status>
	The problem I am calling about is _____.
	    I am afraid the patient is going to arrest.
	
	I have just assessed the patient personally:
	
	Vital signs are: Blood pressure ____/____, Pulse____, Respiration____, and temperature____
	
	I am concerned about the:
	    Blood pressure because it is over 200 or less than 100 or 30 mmHg below usual
	    Pulse because it is over 140 or less than 50
	    Respiration because it is less than 5 or over 40
	    Temperature because it is less than 96 or over 104

B	**Background**
	The patient's mental status is:
	    Alert and oriented to person place and time
	    Confused and cooperative or non-cooperative
	    Agitated or combative
	    Lethargic but conversant and able to swallow
	    Stuporous and not talking clearly and possibly not able to swallow
	    Comatose. Eyes closed. Not responding to stimulation.
	The skin is:
	    Warm and dry
	    Pale
	    Mottled
	    Diaphoretic
	    Extremities are cold
	    Extremities are warm
	The patient is not or is on oxygen.
	    The patient has been on _____ (l/min) or (%) oxygen for _____ minutes (hours)
	    The oximeter is reading ____%
	    The oximeter does not detect a good pulse and is giving erratic readings

A	**Assessment**
	    This is what I think the problem is: \<say what you think is the problem>
	    The problem seems to be cardiac infection neurologic respiratory _____
	    I am not sure what the problem is but the patient is deteriorating.
	    The patient seems to be unstable and may get worse, we need to do something.

R	**Recommendation**
	I suggest or request that you \<say what you would like to see done>.
	    Transfer the patient to critical care.
	    Come to see the patient at this time.
	    Talk to the patient or family about code status.
	    Ask the on-call family practice resident to see the patient now.
	    Ask for a consultant to see the patient now.
	Are any tests needed:
	    Do you need any test like CXR, ABG, EKG, CBC, or BMP?
	    Other?
	If a change in treatment is ordered, then ask:
	    How often do you want vital signs?
	    How long do you expect this problem will last?
	    If the patient does not get better, when would you want us to call again?

● Figure 7.6   SBAR report to physicians about critical situations.

Whether in person or in a phone conversation, document discussions of patient care with other health-care providers. To decrease errors in communication, you can use your concept map to organize the SBAR report of what you will say over the phone to the physician. You must record what was discussed and what was done after the conversation. For example:

> 8/8/01 1500 Pain r/t incision: Dr. Morrow notified per phone Percodan (oxycodone/aspirin) did not relieve pain after 1 hour. Reports pain 9 on 10-point scale. N. DiRenzo, YSU, SN
> 1510 Per order, given 50 mg Demerol IM stat. See MAR (medication administration record). N. DiRenzo, YSU, SN
> 1545 Reports pain 4 on 10-point scale. States "pain much better, but still not gone." N. DiRenzo, YSU, SN

Never write critical comments about another health-care provider or make entries suggesting an error or unsafe practice. Do not write, "Physician made error in the orders." Instead, write "Physician called to clarify." Include in the written statement the objective patient behaviors that relate to the error or unsafe practice if applicable.

In the progress notes, always chart changes in the patient's condition, abnormal test results, and the time that the changes were reported to the physician. Additionally, report threats of legal action or bodily harm from the patient or family toward any member of the health-care team or organization. Record and report to the physician and hospital administrators when the patient displays risks to himself, such as drug or alcohol abuse, or if the patient is refusing treatment or is unwilling to comply with recommendations. Equipment malfunction is also recorded and reported to supervisors.

CHAPTER 7 SUMMARY

Concept care maps are valuable guides for documentation of patient care. Documentation is very important, because it is the legal record of patient care and, in many instances, the basis for financial reimbursement by insurance companies, Medicare, and Medicaid. Good documentation is concise, accurate, complete, legible, timely, logically organized, and confidential. It is a challenge to learn to do it well, but concept care maps will help to remind you of all that must be documented. As the basis of documentation, you will use the diagram, outcomes and interventions, as well as data collected regarding patient responses to interventions to complete standardized forms and narrative notes.

Routine assessments are performed and documented using standardized forms, with specific problems expanded in narrative form using progress notes. The mnemonic PIE is useful to simplify narrative writing: P involves writing about *Problems*, I denotes *Interventions*, and E stands for *Evaluation* of patient responses. You must describe the problem meticulously, describe what you did about the problem, and then describe the patient response to the nursing intervention you performed to alleviate the problem.

Documentation of communication with other health-care providers is extremely important to avoid patient care errors. The concept care map can be used to guide the development of the SBAR to improve the succinct and accurate report to a physician and decrease sentinel events.

LEARNING ACTIVITIES

1. The following are charting excerpts taken from actual medical records. For each entry, what needs to be done to correct it?
   * *By the time he was admitted, his rapid heart had stopped, and he was feeling better.*
   * *Patient has chest pain if she lies on her left side for over a year.*

- *She has had no rigors or shaking chills, but her husband says she was very hot in bed last night.*
- *The patient has been depressed since she began seeing me in 1993.*
- *I have suggested that he loosen his pants before standing, and then, he stands with the help of his wife, they should fall to the floor.*
- *Healthy appearing decrepit 69-year-old male, mentally alert but forgetful.*
- *Patient has left his white blood cells at another hospital.*
- *The patient refused an autopsy.*
- *The patient is tearful and crying constantly. She also appears to be depressed.*
- *Large brown stool ambulating in the hall.*
- *Skin: somewhat pale but present.*
- *Patient has two teenage children but no other abnormalities.*
- *The patient had waffles for breakfast and anorexia for lunch.*
- *She slipped on ice and her legs went in separate directions in early December.*
- *Discharge status: Alive but without permission.*
- *Patient released to the outpatient department without dressing.*
- *The patient expired on the floor uneventfully.*
- *The patient has no past history of suicides.*
- *Since she can't get pregnant without her husband, I thought you would like to work her up.*
- *The patient will need disposition, and therefore we will get Dr. Smith to dispose of him.*

2. Practice writing narrative PIE statements for the concept care map of the diabetic patient. Use Figures 5.1 and 5.2 from Chapter 5.

3. Practice using the concept care map in Figures 5.1 and 5.2 to develop an SBAR.

REFERENCES

1. Nursing's Social Policy Statement, ed 2. American Nurses Association, nurses-books.org, Washington, D.C., 2003.
2. 2006 Comprehensive Accreditation Manual for Hospitals: The Official Handbook. Joint Commission on Accreditation of Healthcare Organizations, Chicago, 2006.
3. Nursing 99 Charting Tips: Easy as PIE. Nursing 99 29(4): 25, 1999 (seminal article).
4. Springhouse: Documentation in Action. Lippincott, Williams and Wilkins, Philadelphia, 2005.
5. Principles for Documentation. American Nurses Association, Silver Spring, MD, 2005.
6. Harman, L. HIPPA: A few years later. Online Journal of Issues in Nursing. Retrieved May 31, 2005, from www.nursingworld.org/ojin/topic27/tpc 27-2.htm
7. Joint Commission on Accreditation of Healthcare Organizations. Root causes of sentinel events. Retrieved November 16, 2005, from http:www.jcaho.org/ accredited+organizations/ambulatory+ care/sentinel+events/root+causes+of+ sentinel+event.htm
8. Institute for Healthcare Improvement. SBAR technique for communication: A situational briefing model. Retrieved September 20, 2005, from http://ihi.org/ IHI/Topics/Patient Safety/SafetyGeneral/ Tools/SBARTechniqueforCommunication ASituationalBriefingModel.htm

AFTER THE CLINICAL DAY IS OVER:
Patient Evaluations, Self-Evaluations, and Grading the Final Concept Care Map

OBJECTIVES

1. Identify standards of nursing performance related to patient care evaluations and performance evaluations.

2. Describe purposes of performance evaluations.

3. Compare formative and summative evaluations.

4. Explain what to do when an error is made.

5. Compare constructive criticism with negative criticism.

6. Analyze criteria for dismissal from clinical.

7. Identify criteria for grading concept care maps.

The clinical day is over, and there is very little left to do. Students spend only about 30 to 60 minutes after leaving the clinical site summarizing patient progress toward goals and outcome objectives and performing self-evaluations of clinical performance. The time is spent reflecting on clinical performance and patient responses to nursing interventions and writing summaries. The primary focus of this chapter is on your professional nursing performance during the clinical day. The American Nurses Association (ANA) has developed standards of professional nursing performance. The first two of these performance standards involve systematic evaluation of the quality and effectiveness of nursing practice and the evaluation of one's own nursing practice.[1]

A very important aspect of a nurse's professional responsibility is self-evaluation of performance. Your self-evaluation must be an accurate perception of your abilities. Your clinical faculty will also evaluate your performance weekly with periodic summary evaluations.

In addition to performing a self-evaluation, you will need to finish evaluation of patient responses and their progress toward objectives, which you started earlier at the clinical site. Think about and record patients' physical and emotional behavioral responses. Consider the extent to which the patient objectives were attained or not, and write about it under the evaluation summary of the patient progress toward the outcome objectives described in Chapter 5. You will also need to finish patient responses to teaching.

This chapter also provides criteria for grading the concept care map. You need to know the criteria that will be used for grading your concept care map so that you can earn an A on your final edition.

Purpose of Performance Evaluations

A performance evaluation is the process of determining how well the nursing student does what is required. Both you and your clinical faculty will evaluate your performance. As the faculty critiques your performance, the purpose is not to blame or shame students. The questions to be addressed with the performance evaluation are: "Do you provide safe and effective care?," "What grade did you earn?," and, by the end of the term, "Should you be promoted to the next level?"[2-4]

Your performance will be compared with established standards that define goals to be attained over time. Each course has expected performance standards that will be stated clearly and in measurable behaviors. The clinical objectives and specific daily objectives of the course are used as standards to evaluate performance.

Performance evaluations are based on those standards and objective criteria, not on personalities or whether a faculty member likes a student. Students must "own" and accept the consequences of their mistakes. Sometimes mistakes lead to a bad grade on a test in a theory course; sometimes they lead to poor patient care or accidental injury to a student. Following are sample objectives for clinical evaluations categorized by nursing process, documentation, and professional qualities.

Clinical Performance Objectives

Identify your strengths and weaknesses for each of the following clinical objectives:

Assessment

1. Prepares each patient profile by gathering complete, relevant information needed to develop a concept care map
   a. Defines medical diagnoses
   b. Defines surgical procedures and diagnostic tests
   c. Defines diagnostic test reports
   d. Defines treatments
   e. Defines medications
   f. Obtains health assessment data from the records

Nursing Diagnoses

1. Develops a concept care map diagram
   a. Identifies physiological, psychological, and educational problems
   b. Prioritizes diagnoses
   c. Correctly categorizes data
   d. Correctly links diagnoses

Planning

1. Develops patient goals, objectives, and nursing interventions
   a. Lists goals and objectives for each diagnosis
   b. Lists nursing interventions to attain objectives
   c. States rationales for interventions

Implementation

1. Provides safe and effective nursing care
   a. Obtains change-of-shift information and integrates on care map
   b. Checks for updated orders at the beginning of the day and throughout the day and integrates on the care map
   c. Organizes time, works in an organized manner, and gets care completed on time
   d. Immediately reports assessment abnormalities and problems to the clinical faculty or to a staff nurse
   e. Keeps bed down and locked with side rails up and call light within patient's reach when not with the patient
   f. Maintains a safe environment by avoiding activities that could potentially put self or others at risk for injury and by using correct protective actions for patients, coworkers, and self
   g. Leaves patient's room neat and clean
   h. Continually checks patient safety and comfort needs throughout clinical day
2. Safely and effectively implements all procedures and treatments
   a. Practices and reviews procedures and treatments prior to clinical
   b. Determines basic-care needs and safely performs all procedures without being reminded (examples: cough and deep breathe, turning, intake and output, range of motion, vital signs, skin care)
   c. Follows standard precautions with all procedures and treatments
   d. Follows hospital and departmental policies with all procedures and treatments
   e. Displays confidence and composure when carrying out procedures and treatments
   f. Prepares patient/family prior to procedures/treatments
   g. Shows respect for privacy needs
   h. Involves family in care of patient
3. Safely and effectively administers medications
   a. Rechecks the medication records each morning for updates
   b. Questions discrepancies in medication records.
   c. Checks for medication allergies on chart and patient armband
   d. Demonstrates knowledge of medications
   e. Accurately calculates medication doses with 100% accuracy
   f. Accurately calculates intravenous flow rates
   g. Assesses the five rights prior to administering any medication
   h. Checks appropriate laboratory work related to medication administration
   i. Evaluates assessment data prior to medication administration
   j. Checks all medications with faculty prior to administration
   k. Uses proper technique when preparing and administering medications
   l. Gives all medications in the allotted time period
4. Safely and effectively teaches and is emotionally supportive to patients and families
   a. Uses the METHOD teaching plan
   b. Provides teaching for patients and family as needed related to METHOD
   c. Demonstrates knowledge of teaching-learning and developmental principles
   d. Answers patient/family's questions and gives explanations in appropriate and understandable terms without causing the patient or family undue anxiety
   e. Provides psycho-social-cultural support for patient and families including the use of touch, humor, empathy, anticipatory guidance, play, relaxation techniques, distraction, reminiscence, and music
5. Communicates effectively
   a. Demonstrates appropriate verbal and nonverbal behaviors in patient/family care

b. Avoids saying or doing anything that could cause undue anxiety for the patient or family

c. Reports off to the faculty and appropriate personnel when leaving for breaks or at the end of clinical

d. Communicates as needed with other health-care providers in planning and carrying out the plan of care

e. Informs the faculty and cover nurse immediately regarding any changes in patient's condition or when any problem is encountered

f. Is pleasant and courteous during all interactions, using therapeutic communication techniques

6. Collaborates with other health-care workers

a. Actively participates as a health-care team member

b. Discusses concept care map with others (faculty, students, staff)

c. Assists other patients at the site in addition to those assigned

d. Interacts effectively with faculty, student, and staff to accomplish objectives

e. Assists other health team members as time permits

f. Actively participates in pre- and post-conferences

Evaluation

1. Evaluates the concept care map

a. Assesses the patient's progress toward objectives

b. Assesses patient's behavioral responses to nursing interventions

c. Modifies the plan of care as needed based on reassessment

2. Evaluates self-performance

a. Objectively assesses self-performance

b. Immediately admits mistakes and takes actions to correct them

c. Accepts constructive criticism without making excuses for behaviors

d. Assumes responsibility for own actions; knows limitations and when to seek guidance

e. Performs weekly, midterm, and final self-evaluations

f. Identifies own strengths and weaknesses

g. Sets own goals and objectives and strives to attain them

h. Seeks appropriate experiences at agencies to meet individual needs

Documentation

1. Documents accurately, concisely, completely, and in a timely manner

a. Records assessment data on appropriate forms (such as flow sheets or progress notes)

b. Documents without being reminded

c. Uses PIE format to document abnormal assessment findings and follow-up actions taken

d. Consults faculty when charting abnormal assessment findings

e. Demonstrates neatness and organization of charting; uses correct terminology, phraseology, and spelling

f. Follows agency policy regarding documentation (such as using only approved abbreviations and black ink only) and corrects errors in charting with one line

Professional Qualities

1. Acts professionally at all times

a. Follows ANA standards of care and standards of nursing performance at all times

b. Follows all policies of the nursing program regarding clinical conduct

c. Updates cardiopulmonary resuscitation test, immunizations, and tuberculosis test yearly

d. Follows the dress code, presenting with professional attire and behavior during clinical and when obtaining assignments

e. Submits written work that is neat, organized, complete, and on time

f. Carefully follows directions

g. Takes the initiative in arranging for make-up of missed written or clinical work
h. Is punctual in reporting to or leaving the clinical agency; when ill, calls the agency and faculty prior to scheduled arrival time
2. Acts ethically at all times
   a. Shows respect for patient and family
   b. Calls patient by name and title
   c. Respects patient's personal space
   d. Maintains confidentiality related to patient information
   e. Follows ANA Code of Ethics for Nurses

Your clinical faculty will use critical incidents, rating scales, or both to help you identify your strengths and weaknesses. Weekly clinical performance appraisal recordings are used to document actual incidents of successful or unsuccessful performance. In using the critical incident approach, you will be asked to list specific actions, reactions, or attributes that were strengths or weaknesses. Two sample clinical performance appraisal assessment forms are shown in Figures 8.1 and 8.2. Faculty will specify the specific behaviors that are expected dependent on course objectives. In Figure 8.1, note that you must complete an accurate self-evaluation and that faculty comments are next to yours. Figure 8.2 is a sample anecdotal note that is completed when a student's performance is not acceptable and the clinical situation is carefully documented and may be placed in the student's academic record.

Constructive Criticism

Criticism is a fact of life and something we all must face. The only way to avoid criticism is to live isolated from other people, but a career in nursing is anything but isolated. We all have had our work, our personalities, and our behaviors criticized at some point. No matter how hard we try, someone is going to be unhappy with us about something; actually, the best any of us can do is to please some of the people some of the time. Sometimes criticism is ungrounded and is

based on a difference of opinion.[5] In this case, one opinion is as good as any other, provided you believe in respecting others' rights to their opinions. In this situation, be assertive and say, "Your opinion is noted. However, I do not agree and plan to continue etc."

Other times, the criticism received is valuable and helpful and thus requires changing behaviors. The valuable and helpful criticism is termed constructive criticism. Constructive criticism is based on incomplete performance of specific behavioral objectives. Its intent is not to shame or blame on a personal level. Specifically, the intent of constructive criticism from your nursing faculty is to give you feedback on your performance and to help you grow into your role as a professional nurse.

Carrying Out Responsibilities and Showing Initiative

As a nursing student, you have many responsibilities that grow with each term in the nursing program. You are expected to perform to the best of your ability and also to take the initiative and look for opportunities to learn new information and skills. For whatever level in nursing you are currently in, there will be specific tasks to perform and specific methods to use in performing them. Once you know your responsibilities, it is up to you to carry them out. If you are unsure of what to do or are afraid of not doing something well, consult with your clinical faculty to get some help. If you do not know how to do something, ask. It is better to admit you do not know something than to have your clinical faculty find out when something is not done. The latter scenario reflects poorly on you and—more seriously—may jeopardize care of the patient.

The fastest way to be dismissed from clinical and possibly even from the nursing program is to jeopardize patient safety. Performance appraisals are used to decide if a student should be dismissed. Not everyone has the ability to be a nurse. Following are some samples of unacceptable clinical behaviors, taken from the Youngstown State University Department of Nursing Undergraduate Student Handbook[6]:

WEEKLY CLINICAL SELF EVALUATION   Student _____

Date of Clinical _____

Patient Initials: _____ Age: ____ Medical Diagnosis(es) _____

Allergies: _____   **Faculty Comments**

ASSESSMENT–Prepares each patient profile by gathering complete information needed to develop a care map. Defines medical diagnoses, surgical procedures, diagnostic tests, treatments, medications, physical assessment.
STUDENT COMMENTS
YOUR STRENGTHS:

YOUR WEAKNESSES AND REMEDY TO IMPROVE:

NURSING DIAGNOSIS(es)–Brings to clinical each week a concept care map and identifies physiological and psycho-social problems, correctly categorizes data on the map, prioritizes problems, links problems and labels diagnoses.
STUDENT COMMENTS
YOUR STRENGTHS:

YOUR WEAKNESSES AND REMEDY TO IMPROVE:

PLANNING–Comes prepared to clinical with a developed care map that include goals, objectives, and interventions; and states rationales for interventions. Collaborates with staff, faculty, and students in planning coordinated nursing care. Participates in clincal pre and post conferences.
STUDENT COMMENTS
YOUR STRENGTHS:

YOUR WEAKNESSES AND REMEDY TO IMPROVE:

IMPLEMENTATION Safely performs procedures and medication administration. Organizes time, works in an organized manner, and gets care completed on time. Uses therapeutic communication techniques such as touch, humor, empathy, anticipatory guidance, relaxation techniques, distraction, reminiscence, and music to reduce anxiety. Interacts effectively with staff, faculty, and other students.
STUDENT COMMENTS
YOUR STRENGTHS:

YOUR WEAKNESSES AND REMEDY TO IMPROVE:

Patient EVALUATION: Assesses patient's progress toward objectives and responses to nursing interventions and modifies the plan as needed. Informs the faculty and cover nurse immediately regarding any changes in the patient condition or when any problem is encountered.
STUDENT COMMENTS
YOUR STRENGTHS:

YOUR WEAKNESSES AND REMEDY TO IMPROVE:

Self-EVALUATION: Admits mistakes and takes actions to correct them, accepts constructive criticism, seeks out experiences, know limitations, and seeks guidance when needed.
STUDENT COMMENTS
YOUR STRENGTHS:

YOUR WEAKNESSES AND REMEDY TO IMPROVE:

DOCUMENTATION: Documents accurately, concisely, completely, and in a timely manner. Consults faculty before documenting abnormal findings. Follows agency policies regarding documentation.
STUDENT COMMENTS
YOUR STRENGTHS:

YOUR WEAKNESSES AND REMEDY TO IMPROVE:

PROFESSIONAL QUALITIES: Follows ANA standards of care and code of ethics, follows the dress codes and all policies of the nursing program regarding clinical conduct. Is always on time and comes with prepared care plan.
STUDENT COMMENTS
YOUR STRENGTHS:

YOUR WEAKNESSES AND REMEDY TO IMPROVE:

● Figure 8.1   Hospital weekly objectives and clinical self-evaluation/faculty evaluation.

Youngstown State University
Bachelor Degree Program in Nursing

Nursing_____ – _____
Semester, 20 ____

Anecdotal Note

Name of Student: _____ Date: _____

The Situation

_____
_____
_____
_____

Description of Student's Actions

_____
_____
_____
_____

Instructor's Evaluation

_____
_____
_____
_____

Instructor's Signature: _____

● Figure 8.2   Anecdotal note.

Dismissal for Unacceptable Clinical Behavior Policy

The Department of Nursing reserves the right to dismiss a student from the program &/or Clinical who demonstrates unacceptable clinical behaviors that include, but are not limited to:

1. Failure to pick up a clinical assignment or inadequate preparation for clinical experience;

2. Attending clinical experiences under the influence of drugs and/or alcohol;
3. Refusing to care for an assigned patient based on patient's characteristics; e.g., race, culture, religious beliefs, or diagnosis;
4. Participating in acts of omission or commission in the care of patients, such as physical abuse; placing the patient in a hazardous position, condition, or circumstance; mental/emotional abuse;

5. Disrupting of patient care or unit functioning related to poor interpersonal relationships with agency health team members, peers, or faculty;

6. Demonstrating behavior that affects one or more parameters of safe clinical practice and/or jeopardizes the well-being of the patient, patient families, health team members, peers, or faculty;

7. Documenting dishonestly, breaching patient confidentiality, solicitation of patient for services leading to personal gain, and other behaviors as listed under Professionalism Category of the Clinical Evaluation Tool;

8. Failing to adhere to the Ohio Board of Nursing Rules Regulating the Practice of Nursing as of February 1, 2004, 4723-5-12.

   ▶ A student shall report and document nursing assessments or observations, the care provided by the student for the patient, and the patient's response to that care;

   ▶ A student shall accurately and timely report to the appropriate practitioner errors in or deviations from the prescribed regimen of care;

   ▶ A student shall not falsify any patient record or any other document prepared or utilized in the course of, or in conjunction with, nursing practice;

   ▶ A student shall implement measures to promote a safe environment for each patient;

   ▶ A student shall delineate, establish, and maintain professional boundaries with each patient;

   ▶ At all times when a student is providing direct nursing care to a patient the student shall:

      (a) Provide privacy during examination or treatment and in the care of personal or bodily needs; and

      (b) Treat each patient with courtesy, respect, and with full recognition of dignity and individuality

   ▶ A student shall not:

      (a) Engage in behavior that causes or may cause physical, verbal, mental or emotional abuse to a patient; or

      (b) Engage in behavior toward a patient that may reasonably be interpreted as physical, verbal, mental or emotional abuse

   ▶ A student shall not misappropriate a patient's property or:

      (a) Engage in behavior to seek or obtain personal gain at the patient's expense;

      (b) Engage in behavior that may reasonably be interpreted as behavior to seek or obtain personal gain at the patient's expense;

      (c) Engage in behavior that constitutes inappropriate involvement in the patient's personal relationships; or

      (d) Engage in behavior that may reasonably be interpreted as inappropriate involvement in the patient's personal relationships

For the purpose of this paragraph, the patient is always presumed incapable of giving free, full, or informed consent to the behaviors by the student set forth in this paragraph.

   ▶ A student shall not:

      (a) Engage in sexual conduct with a patient;

      (b) Engage in conduct that may reasonably be interpreted as sexual;

      (c) Engage in any verbal behavior that is seductive or sexually demeaning to a patient; or

      (d) Engage in verbal behavior that may reasonably be interpreted as seductive or sexually demeaning to a patient

For the purpose of this paragraph, the patient is always presumed incapable of giving free, full, or informed consent to sexual activity with the student.

The student's behavior must demonstrate competency by responsible preparation, implementation, and documentation of the nursing care of patients. In addition, the student's behavior must be respectful of all individuals (patient, patient's family, health team members, and self) according to the AHA Patient's Bill of Rights, the ANA Standard of Care, and the ANA Code for Nurses.

Due Process

A student who exhibits unacceptable clinical behavior and/or violates student conduct requirements set forth by the Ohio Board of Nursing will be given a verbal and written performance report by the clinical faculty member. The performance report becomes part of the student's academic file.

The faculty member will notify the AP&G Committee of the student's conduct, violation and/or unacceptable behavior for further consideration. The AP&G Committee will consider documented evidence from the student, faculty, or health care team members when making recommendations regarding continuation of the student's participation in the program and/or clinical. The AP&G recommendation will be presented to the General Faculty and/or Chairperson of the Department of Nursing for the final decision. The student will be notified of the decision, in writing, by the AP&G Committee.

Clinical Evaluations: Formative and Summative

Clinical faculty expects students to be in a state of continuous development throughout the nursing program and for students to make increasing contributions to the clinical care of patients. There are links between performance evaluation, professional growth and development, and the rewards of providing excellent care.[7-9] Faculty and students give feedback to each other in order to evaluate the student's performance, professional growth, and development. The focus is on behaviors and skills. Students and faculty alike receive rewards when the care of patients is done well. Faculty members are very proud of students who receive compliments from both the patients and staff for the good job they are doing or have done, and students are proud of themselves, too. The cycle of performance, evaluation, professional growth, and reward is detailed in Figure 8.3.

THE CYCLE OF PERFORMANCE, EVALUATION, PROFESSIONAL GROWTH, AND REWARDS

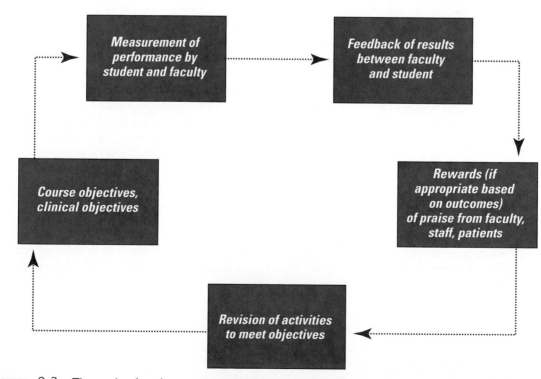

● Figure 8.3   The cycle of performance, evaluation, professional growth, and rewards.

Formative Evaluations

Start each term by reviewing specific clinical objectives that you will need to meet in order to complete the course. It is very important for you to be aware of what is expected of you. Then weekly, you and your faculty will select experiences to meet those objectives. For example, during the term just completed, you did not have time to perfect your injection skills, so you ask your faculty to arrange some additional experiences to develop this skill while you still meet current course objectives.

Weekly, there will be ongoing progress reviews and guidance from your clinical faculty. Students do weekly self-evaluations of strengths and weaknesses with regard to attaining the course objectives. You must objectively write down what you have done well or what needs improvement. Be sure to include any feedback from your faculty in your assessment. Faculty want to see on a weekly basis that what they are telling you is being performed. When you give your self-evaluation to the faculty, they will write their comments. The intent is to monitor behaviors and skills closely because human lives are at stake. It is very important that you know weekly what your clinical faculty member thinks of your performance.

Nurses have awesome responsibilities for the safe care of patients, and you and your faculty are working together closely to prevent catastrophic mistakes from occurring. Faculty and students recognize that mistakes will be made, but avoiding a catastrophic mistake is the primary objective.

Summative Evaluations

Each clinical course also entails summative evaluations. Usually at midterm and at the end of the term, you and your clinical faculty will have a summative formal conference to review your progress toward meeting course objectives. At midterm, establish individualized performance objectives to accomplish by the end of the term. With weekly formative evaluations, nothing at the summative review should come as a surprise. You and your faculty will review how you have done relative to the agreed-upon objectives over time. If problems in attaining objectives occur, there must be a discussion about why the objectives have not been met, and a new plan needs to be developed for meeting the objectives within the time constraints of the term. Specific steps to take for improvement are decided upon.

Whether the evaluation is formative or summative, there are some basic principles of receiving an evaluation to always remember and do.[9] These include:

1. Consider all your constructive criticism feedback as having been given with helpful intent.
2. Listen to your faculty's perspective, and avoid excuses.
3. Ask for clarification, and ask for examples of any inappropriate behavior.
4. Check with your clinical faculty for mutual understanding.
5. Ask for help and support in the areas of future growth.

Now You've Blown It: Making Mistakes

Perhaps you have recapped a contaminated needle, forgot to aspirate, or forgot to wear gloves when doing a subcutaneous injection and there was some bleeding at the site. Now what? First, remember that everyone makes mistakes because no one is perfect. It is part of human nature to make mistakes. You must accept responsibility and be straightforward: "I really blew it by not aspirating." Admit your mistake; do not make excuses because doing so will indicate that you cannot accept responsibility for what you have done. Here is a sample excuse from student to faculty: "You made me so nervous by being in the room with me that I forgot to aspirate." Your faculty does not want to hear excuses, and they will lose respect for you if you use them. Blaming your faculty for your lack of performance is certainly an avoidance of responsibility.

Suppose the faculty member was not present to see the mistake. For example, you neglect to get a patient up for ambulation in the morning because the patient said he was too weak to move. The staff nurse goes to check the patient, asks him if he has walked yet, finds out he has not, and irately tells you that patient must be walked immediately. Do you tell your faculty member about it or not? Maybe the faculty member will not find out, and you can cover it up. Honesty and integrity are paramount to safe and effective nursing care. It is much better for you to tell your faculty about your error in judgment than to let the clinical faculty find out about it from someone else. Faculty want to hear about the error from you directly, because it demonstrates that you take responsibility by owning up to your mistakes. If the faculty thinks that you are purposely covering up an error, it means that you cannot be trusted. A student covering up mistakes is acting unethically because it is dishonest.

Second, do not beat yourself up publicly or privately about mistakes. It is unhealthy to engage in self-recrimination or statements such as, "I'm stupid and will never make a good nurse." A better way to think is, "I'm intelligent, but I made a mistake that I will never make again." Focus on the behavior that you need to

improve. You need to learn and grow from the mistake. Analyze what went wrong, solve the problem, and do not repeat the error.[10]

Grading Concept Care Maps: How to Get an "A"

Figure 8.4 contains a sample care plan grading criteria form for the concept care map. For each criterion, one point is given if you do a good job summarizing information, a half point for some correct information and some incorrect or missing information, and zero points for a poor job on the information. These sample care plan criteria are useful for a medical-surgical hospitalized patient. Criteria will vary depending on the type of clinical setting and the level of the course in the curriculum. Good luck with concept care maps....it takes much time and effort to learn to organize and provide patient care, but your efforts will bring many satisfying rewards, and you will become an excellent nurse!

CHAPTER 8 SUMMARY

You need ongoing exchanges with clinical faculty about performance for successful growth through constructive criticism and evaluation. Both the faculty and you sometimes need to say hard things, although in a respectful manner by being open and honest, and you should trust each other to have best interests in mind. Avoid becoming defensive or argumentative; stick with the facts. You will be receiving regular, constructive, and candid feedback from your clinical faculty. Your faculty will direct you where to go for assistance as needed (for example, the references to review or the skills laboratory for further practice, the mathematics center, or the writing center).

However, you alone must take responsibility for your own development. You must seek out learning experiences to develop yourself in ways that support the achievement of outstanding nursing care.

LEARNING ACTIVITIES

1. Compare course objectives from two sequential clinical nursing courses. Describe differences in focus and expectations.

2. Analyze clinical site behavioral objectives for an agency you will use as a clinical site, and give examples of behaviors that may be considered strengths and weaknesses.

3. Review your school's dismissal policy, and compare it with the sample in the chapter.

4. Use the grading guide to grade a concept care map you have developed.

ANA Standard I Assessment

General Survey	0 1/2 1
Health Assessment Data Base (Chapter 2 p.)	0 1/2 1
Medical Diagnoses	0 1/2 1
Surgical Procedures	0 1/2 1
Medications	0 1/2 1
Laboratory	0 1/2 1
Skin Assessment Complete (Chapter 3 p.)	0 1/2 1
Falls Assessment Complete (Chapter 3 p.)	0 1/2 1
Glasgow Coma Scale (Chapter 3 p.)	0 1/2 1
Psychosocial Assessment (Chapter 6 p.)	0 1/2 1
Pain Assessment (Chapter 3 p.)	0 1/2 1

ANA Standard II Nursing Problem Analyses-Steps 1-3 Map-Chapter 3

Identifies Physiological Problems	0 1/2 1
Identifies Psychological Problems	0 1/2 1
Identifies Education Needs	0 1/2 1
Correctly Links Problems	0 1/2 1
Correctly Identifies Reason for Health Care (central box)	0 1/2 1
Key Assessments (central box)	0 1/2 1
Abnormal Assessment Data in correct boxes	0 1/2 1
Medications Categorized in correct boxes	0 1/2 1
Treatments Categorized in correct boxes	0 1/2 1
Diagnostic Tests in correct boxes	0 1/2 1
Correctly Prioritizes Problems	0 1/2 1
Correctly Labels Nursing Diagnoses (NANDA)	0 1/2 1

ANA Standards III, IV, V, Planning-Steps 4 Chapter 4

Lists goals for all

Physical Problems	0 1/2 1
Psychosocial Problems	0 1/2 1

Lists objectives for all

Physical Problems	0 1/2 1
Psychosocial Problems	0 1/2 1

Lists all nursing interventions to attain objectives

Assessments to be Performed	0 1/2 1
Communication/Psychological Interventions	0 1/2 1
Physiological Interventions	0 1/2 1
Nursing Interventions provide for patient/family participation	0 1/2 1

ANA Standards VII & VIII Evaluation-Step 5 Chapter 5

Evaluates patients behavioral responses to nursing interventions for

1 Priority physical nursing diagnosis	0 1/2 1
1 Priority psychosocial nursing diagnosis	0 1/2 1

Under impressions, evaluate patient progress toward

Outcome objectives for

1 priority physical diagnosis	0 1/2 1
1 priority psychosocial diagnosis	0 1/2 1
Total Points	_/35 =_

● Figure 8.4 Grading criteria concept map care plan evaluation.

REFERENCES

1. Nursing's Social Policy Statement, ed 2. American Nurses Association, nurses-books.org, Washington, D.C., 2003.
2. Clardy, A: Managing Human Resources: Exercise, Experiments, and Applications Workbook. Lawrence Erlbaum Associates, Inc. Mahwah, NJ, 1996.
3. Pynes, JE: Human Resources Management for Public and Nonprofit Organizations, ed 2. Jossey-Bass Publishers, San Francisco, 2004.
4. Arthur, D: Managing Human Resources in Small and Mid-Sized Companies, ed 2. American Management Association, New York, 1995.
5. Carlson, R: Don't Sweat the Small Stuff at Work. Hyperion, New York, 1999.
6. Youngstown State University Department of Nursing Undergraduate Student Handbook, 2006.
7. Gratton, L, et al: Strategic Human Resource Management, ed 4. Oxford University Press, New York, 2005.
8. Carr, C: The New Manager's Survival Manual: All the Skills You Need for Success. John Wiley and Sons, New York, 1995.
9. Mabey, C, et al: Human Resource Management: A Strategic Introduction, ed 2. Blackwell, Malden, MA, 1998.
10. Komisarjevsky, C, and Komisarjevsky, R: Peanut Butter and Jelly Management: Tales From Parenthood, Lessons for Managers. American Management Association, New York, 2004.

Nursing Diagnoses Arranged by Maslow's Hierarchy of Needs

Physiological Needs

Activity Intolerance
Activity Intolerance, Risk for
Airway Clearance, Ineffective
Aspiration, Risk for
Breastfeeding, Effective
Breastfeeding, Ineffective
Breastfeeding, Interrupted
Breathing Pattern, Ineffective
Cardiac Output, Decreased
Confusion, Acute
Confusion, Chronic
Constipation
Constipation, Perceived
Constipation, Risk of
Dentition, Impaired
Diarrhea
Environmental Interpretation
    Syndrome, Impaired
Fatigue
Fluid Volume, Deficient
Fluid Volume, Risk for Deficient
Fluid Volume, Excessive
Fluid Volume, Risk for Imbalance
Gas Exchange, Impaired
Hyperthermia
Hypothermia
Incontinence, Bowel
Incontinence, Functional
Incontinence, Reflex
Incontinence, Risk for Urge
Incontinence, Stress
Incontinence, Total
Incontinence, Urge
Infant Behavior, Disorganized

Infant Behavior, Readiness for Enhanced
    Organized
Infant Behavior, Risk for Disorganized
Infant Feeding Pattern, Ineffective
Intracranial, Decreased Adaptive
    Capacity
Memory, Impaired
Mobility, Impaired Bed
Mobility, Impaired Physical
Mobility, Impaired Wheelchair
Nausea
Nutrition, Imbalanced: Less Than Body
    Requirements
Nutrition, Imbalanced: More Than Body
    Requirements
Nutrition, Imbalanced: Risk for More
    Than Body Requirements
Oral Mucous Membranes, Impaired
Pain, Acute
Pain, Chronic
Protection, Ineffective
Self-Care Deficit, Bathing/Hygiene
Self-Care Deficit, Dressing/Grooming
Self-Care Deficit, Feeding
Self-Care Deficit, Toileting
Sensory Perception, Disturbed (Specify)
    (Visual, Auditory, Kinesthetic,
    Gustatory, Tactile, Olfactory)
Sexual Dysfunction
Sexuality Pattern, Ineffective
Skin Integrity, Impaired
Skin Integrity, Impaired, Risk for
Sleep Deprivation
Sleep Pattern, Disturbed
Surgical Recovery, Delayed
Swallowing, Impaired
Temperature, Risk for Imbalanced Body

Thermoregulation, Ineffective
Thought Process, Disturbed
Tissue Integrity, Impaired
Tissue Perfusion, Ineffective (Specify) (Renal,
    Cerebral, Cardiopulmonary, Gastrointestinal,
    Peripheral)
Transfer Ability, Impaired
Urinary Elimination, Impaired
Urinary Retention
Ventilation, Impaired Spontaneous
Ventilatory Weaning Response, Dysfunctional
Walking, Impaired

Safety and Security Needs

Communication, Impaired Verbal
Death Anxiety
Disuse Syndrome, Risk for
Dysreflexia
Dysreflexia, Risk for Autonomic
Falls, Risk for
Fear
Grieving, Anticipatory
Grieving, Dysfunctional
Growth, Risk for Disproportional
Health Maintenance, Ineffective
Home Maintenance Management, Impaired
Infection, Risk for
Injury, Risk for
Knowledge, Deficient
Latex Allergy
Latex Allergy, Risk for
Perioperative Positioning Injury, Risk for
Peripheral Neurovascular Dysfunction, Risk for
Poisoning, Risk for
Sorrow, Chronic
Suffocation, Risk for
Therapeutic Regimen: Community, Ineffective
    Management of
Therapeutic Regimen: Families, Ineffective
    Management of
Therapeutic Regimen: Individual, Ineffective
    Management of
Trauma, Risk for
Unilateral Neglect
Wandering

Love and Belonging Needs

Adult Failure to Thrive
Anxiety

Caregiver Role Strain
Caregiver Role Strain, Risk for
Family Coping: Compromised, Ineffective
Family Coping: Disabling, Ineffective
Family Coping: Readiness for Enhanced
Family Processes, Interrupted
Loneliness, Risk for
Parent/Infant/Child Attachment, Risk
    for Impaired
Parental Role Conflict
Parenting, Deficient
Parenting, Deficient, Risk for
Relocation Stress Syndrome
Social Interaction, Impaired
Social Isolation

Self-Esteem

Adjustment, Impaired
Alcoholism, Altered Family Process
Body Image Disturbed
Community Coping, Ineffective
Community Coping, Readiness for
    Enhanced
Coping, Defensive
Coping, Ineffective Individual
Decisional Conflict
Denial, Ineffective
Diversional Activity Deficient
Hopelessness
Noncompliance
Identity, Disturbed Personal
Post-Trauma Syndrome
Post-Trauma Syndrome, Risk for
Powerlessness
Powerlessness, Risk for
Rape-Trauma Syndrome
Rape-Trauma Syndrome: Compound
    Reaction
Rape-Trauma Syndrome: Silent Reaction
Relocation Stress Syndrome: Risk for
Role Performance, Ineffective
Self-Esteem, Chronic Low
Self-Esteem, Situational Low
Self-Esteem: Situational Low (Risk for)
Self-Esteem Disturbance
Self-Mutilation
Self-Mutilation, Risk for
Suicide, Risk for
Violence: Self-Directed or Directed at Others,
    Risk for

Self-Actualization Needs

Effective Management of Therapeutic Regimen
Energy Field Disturbed
Growth and Development, Delayed

Delayed Development, Risk for
Health-Seeking Behaviors
Spiritual Well-Being, Readiness for
    Enhanced
Spiritual Distress
Spiritual Distress, Risk for

Nursing Diagnoses Arranged by Gordon's Functional Health Patterns*

Health Perception–Health Management Pattern

Contamination
Disturbed energy field
Effective therapeutic regimen
  management
Health-seeking behaviors (specify)
Ineffective community therapeutic
  regimen management
Ineffective family therapeutic regimen
  management
Ineffective health maintenance
Ineffective protection
Ineffective therapeutic regimen
  management
Noncompliance (specify)
Readiness for enhanced immunization
  status
Readiness for enhanced therapeutic
  regimen management
Risk for exposure to contamination
Risk for falls
Risk for infection
Risk for injury (trauma) [this refers
  to two Nursing Diagnoses]
Risk for perioperative positioning
  injury
Risk for poisoning
Risk for suffocation
Sudden infant death syndrome

Nutritional-Metabolic Pattern

Adult failure to thrive
Deficient fluid volume
Effective breastfeeding
Excess fluid volume
Hyperthermia
Hypothermia
Imbalanced nutrition: less than body
  requirements
Imbalanced nutrition: more than body
  requirements
Impaired dentition
Impaired oral mucous membrane
Impaired skin integrity
Impaired swallowing
Impaired tissue integrity (specify type)
Ineffective breastfeeding
Ineffective infant feeding pattern
Ineffective thermoregulation
Interrupted breastfeeding
Latex allergy response
Nausea
Readiness for enhanced fluid balance
Readiness for enhanced nutrition
Risk for aspiration
Risk for deficient fluid volume
Risk for imbalanced body temperature
Risk for imbalanced fluid volume
Risk for imbalanced nutrition: more
  than body requirements

*Modified by Marjory Gordon, 2007, with permission.

Risk for impaired liver function
Risk for impaired skin integrity
Risk for latex allergy response
Risk for unstable blood glucose

Elimination Pattern

Bowel incontinence
Constipation
Diarrhea
Functional urinary incontinence
Impaired urinary elimination
Overflow urinary incontinence
Perceived constipation
Readiness for enhanced urinary
    elimination
Reflex urinary incontinence
Risk for constipation
Risk for urge urinary incontinence
Stress urinary incontinence
Total incontinence
Urge urinary incontinence
Urinary retention

Activity-Exercise Pattern

Activity intolerance
Autonomic dysreflexia
Decreased cardiac output
Decreased intracranial adaptive capacity
Deficient diversional activity
Delayed growth and development
Delayed surgical recovery
Disorganized infant behavior
Dysfunctional ventilatory weaning response
Fatigue
Impaired spontaneous ventilation
Impaired bed mobility
Impaired gas exchange
Impaired home maintenance
Impaired physical mobility
Impaired transfer ability
Impaired walking
Impaired wheelchair mobility
Ineffective airway clearance
Ineffective breathing pattern
Ineffective tissue perfusion (specify)
Readiness for enhanced organized infant
    behavior

Readiness for enhanced self care
Risk for delayed development
Risk for disorganized infant behavior
Risk for disproportionate growth
Risk for activity intolerance
Risk for autonomic dysreflexia
Risk for disuse syndrome
Risk for peripheral neurovascular dysfunction
Sedentary lifestyle
Self-care deficit (specify: bathing/hygiene,
    dressing/grooming, feeding, toileting)
Wandering

Sleep-Rest Pattern

Disturbed sleep pattern
Readiness for enhanced sleep
Sleep deprivation

Cognitive-Perceptual Pattern

Acute confusion
Acute pain
Chronic confusion
Chronic pain
Decisional conflict (specify)
Deficient knowledge (specify)
Disturbed sensory perception (specify)
Disturbed thought processes
Impaired environmental interpretation
    syndrome
Impaired memory
Readiness for enhanced comfort
Readiness for enhanced decision-making
Readiness for enhanced knowledge (specify)
Risk for acute confusion
Unilateral neglect

Self-Perception–Self-Concept Pattern

Anxiety
Body image disturbed
Chronic low self-esteem
Death anxiety
Disturbed personal identity
Fear
Hopelessness

Powerlessness
Readiness for enhanced hope
Readiness for enhanced power
Readiness for enhanced self-concept
Risk for compromised human dignity
Risk for loneliness
Risk for violence, self-directed
Risk for powerlessness
Risk for situational low self-esteem
Situational low self-esteem

Role-Relationship Pattern

Anticipatory grieving
Caregiver role strain
Chronic sorrow
Dysfunctional family processes:
    alcoholism
Dysfunctional grieving
Impaired parenting
Impaired social interaction
Impaired verbal communication
Ineffective role performance
Interrupted family processes
Parental role conflict
Readiness for enhanced communication
Readiness for enhanced family processes
Readiness for enhanced parenting
Relocation stress syndrome
Risk for caregiver role strain
Risk for dysfunctional grieving
Risk for impaired parent/infant/child
    attachment
Risk for impaired parenting
Risk for relocation stress syndrome
Risk for violence directed at others
Social isolation

Sexuality-Reproductive

Ineffective sexuality pattern
Rape-trauma syndrome
Rape-trauma syndrome: compound reaction
Rape-trauma syndrome: silent reaction
Sexual dysfunction

Coping-Stress Tolerance Pattern

Compromised family coping
Defensive coping
Disabled family coping
Impaired adjustment
Ineffective community coping
Ineffective coping
Ineffective denial
Post-trauma syndrome
Readiness for enhanced community coping
Readiness for enhanced coping
Readiness for enhanced family coping
Risk for post-trauma syndrome
Risk for self-mutilation
Risk for suicide
Self-mutilation
Stress overload

Value-Belief Pattern

Impaired religiosity
Moral distress
Readiness for enhanced religiosity
Readiness for enhanced spiritual well-being
Risk for impaired religiosity
Risk for spiritual distress
Spiritual distress

Nursing Diagnoses Arranged by Doenges & Moorhouse's Diagnostic Divisions*

Activity/Rest

Activity intolerance
Activity intolerance, risk for
Disuse Syndrome, risk for
Diversional Activity, deficient
Fatigue
Insomnia
Mobility, impaired bed
Mobility, impaired wheelchair
Sleep Deprivation
Sleep, readiness for enhanced
Transfer Ability, impaired
Walking, impaired

Circulation

Autonomic Dysreflexia
Autonomic Dysreflexia, risk for
Cardiac Output, decreased
Intracranial adaptive capacity, decreased
Tissue Perfusion, ineffective, (specify type: cerebral, cardiopulmonary, renal, gastrointestinal, peripheral)

Ego Integrity

Anxiety [specify level]
Anxiety, death

Body Image, disturbed
Conflict, decisional (specify)
Coping, defensive
Coping, ineffective
Decision-making, readiness for enhanced
Denial, ineffective
Energy Field, disturbed
Fear (specify)
Grieving
Grieving, complicated
Grieving, risk for complicated
Hope, readiness for enhanced
Hopelessness
Human Dignity, risk for compromised
Moral Distress
Personal Identity, disturbed
Post-Trauma Syndrome
Post-Trauma Syndrome, risk for
Power, readiness for enhanced
Powerlessness
Powerlessness, risk for
Rape-Trauma Syndrome
Rape-Trauma Syndrome: compound reaction
Rape-Trauma Syndrome: silent reaction
Relocation Stress Syndrome
Relocation Stress Syndrome, risk for
Self-concept, readiness for enhanced
Self-Esteem, chronic low
Self-Esteem, situational low
Self-Esteem, risk for situational low
Sorrow, chronic

*Modified by Doenges & Moorhouse, 2007, with permission.

Spiritual Distress
Spiritual Distress, risk for
Spiritual Well-Being, readiness for enhanced

Elimination

Bowel Incontinence
Constipation
Constipation, perceived
Constipation, risk for
Diarrhea
Urinary Elimination, impaired
Urinary Elimination, readiness for enhanced
Urinary Incontinence, functional
Urinary Incontinence, overflow
Urinary Incontinence, reflex
Urinary Incontinence, stress
Urinary Incontinence, total
Urinary Incontinence, urge
Urinary Incontinence, risk for urge
Urinary Retention [acute/chronic]

Food/Fluid

Breastfeeding, effective
Breastfeeding, ineffective
Breastfeeding, interrupted
Dentition, impaired
Failure to Thrive, adult
Fluid balance, readiness for enhanced
[Fluid Volume, deficient (hyper/hypotonic)]
Fluid Volume, deficient [isotonic]
Fluid Volume excess
Fluid Volume, risk for deficient
Fluid Volume, risk for imbalanced
Glucose, risk for unstable level
Infant Feeding Pattern, ineffective
Liver, risk for impaired function
Nausea
Nutrition: less than body requirements,
    imbalanced
Nutrition: more than body requirements,
    imbalanced
Nutrition: risk for more than body
    requirements, imbalanced
Nutrition: readiness for enhanced
Oral Mucous Membrane, impaired
Swallowing, impaired

Hygiene

Self-Care deficit: bathing/hygiene
Self-Care deficit: dressing/grooming
Self-Care deficit: feeding
Self-Care deficit: toileting
Self-Care, readiness for enhanced

Neurosensory

Confusion, acute
Confusion, risk for acute
Confusion, chronic
Infant Behavior, disorganized
Infant Behavior, risk for disorganized
Infant Behavior, readiness for enhanced
    organized
Memory, impaired
Peripheral Neurovascular dysfunction, risk for
Sensory Perception, disturbed (specify: visual,
    auditory, kinesthetic, gustatory, tactile,
    olfactory)
Thought Processes, disturbed
Unilateral Neglect

Pain/Discomfort

Comfort, readiness for enhanced
Pain, acute
Pain, chronic

Respiration

Airway Clearance, ineffective
Aspiration, risk for
Breathing Pattern, ineffective
Gas Exchange, impaired
Ventilation, impaired spontaneous
Ventilatory Weaning Response, dysfunctional

Safety

Allergy response, latex
Allergy response, risk for latex
Body Temperature, risk for imbalanced
Contamination

Contamination, risk for
Death Syndrome, risk for sudden infant
Environmental Interpretation Syndrome,
    impaired
Falls, risk for
Health Behavior, risk prone
Health Maintenance, ineffective
Home Maintenance, impaired
Hyperthermia
Hypothermia
Immunization status, readiness
    for enhanced
Infection, risk for
Injury, risk for
Mobility, impaired physical
Perioperative Positioning, risk for
Poisoning, risk for
Protection, ineffective
Self-Mutilation
Self-Mutilation, risk for
Skin Integrity, impaired
Skin Integrity, risk for impaired
Stress overload
Suffocation, risk for
Suicide, risk for
Surgical Recovery, delayed
Thermoregulation, ineffective
Tissue Integrity, impaired
Trauma, risk for
Violence, [actual/] risk for other-directed
Violence, [actual/] risk for self-directed
Wandering [specify sporadic or continual]

Sexuality

Sexual Dysfunction
Sexuality Pattern, ineffective

Social Interaction

Attachment, risk for impaired
    parent/infant/child

Caregiver Role Strain
Caregiver Role Strain, risk for
Communication, impaired verbal
Communication, readiness for enhanced
Coping, ineffective community
Coping, readiness for enhanced community
Coping, compromised family
Coping, disabled family
Coping, readiness for enhanced family
Family Processes, dysfunctional: alcoholism
Family Processes, interrupted
Family Processes, readiness for enhanced
Loneliness, risk for
Parental Role Conflict
Parenting, impaired
Parenting, readiness for enhanced
Parenting, risk for impaired
Role Performance, ineffective
Social Interaction, impaired
Social Isolation

Teaching/Learning

Development, risk for delayed
Growth & Development, delayed
Growth, risk for disproportionate
Health-Seeking Behaviors (specify)
Knowledge, deficient [Learning Need]
    (specify)
Knowledge of (specify), readiness for
    enhanced
Noncompliance [Adherence,
    ineffective] (specify)
Therapeutic Regimen management:
    ineffective community
Therapeutic Regimen management:
    ineffective family
Therapeutic Regimen management:
    effective
Therapeutic Regimen management:
    ineffective
Therapeutic Regimen management:
    readiness for enhanced

North American Nursing Diagnosis Association's (NANDA) Nursing Diagnosis Categories

Activity Intolerance [specify level]
Activity Intolerance, risk for
Airway Clearance, ineffective
Allergy Response, latex
Allergy response, latex, risk for
Anxiety [specify level]
Anxiety, death
Aspiration, risk for
Attachment, risk for impaired parent/infant/child
Autonomic Dysreflexia
Autonomic Dysreflexia, risk for
Blood Sugar, risk for unstable
Body Image, disturbed
Body Temperature, risk for imbalanced
Bowel Incontinence
Breastfeeding, effective
Breastfeeding, ineffective
Breastfeeding, interrupted
Breathing Pattern, ineffective
Cardiac Output, decreased
Caregiver Role Strain
Caregiver Role Strain, risk for
Comfort, readiness for enhanced
Communication, impaired verbal
Communication, readiness for enhanced
Conflict, parental role
Confusion, acute
Confusion, risk for acute
Confusion, chronic
Constipation
Constipation, perceived
Constipation, risk for

Contamination
Contamination, risk for
Coping, defensive
Coping, ineffective
Coping, readiness for enhanced
Coping, ineffective community
Coping, readiness for enhanced community
Coping, compromised family
Coping, disabled family
Coping, readiness for enhanced family
Death Syndrome, risk for sudden infant
Decisional Conflict (specify)
Denial, ineffective
Dentition, impaired
Decision-Making, readiness for enhanced
Development, risk for delayed
Diarrhea
Disuse Syndrome, risk for
Diversional Activity, deficient
Energy Field, disturbed (revised)
Environmental Interpretation Syndrome, impaired
Failure to Thrive, adult
Falls, risk for
Family Processes: alcoholism, dysfunctional
Family Processes, interrupted
Family Processes, readiness for enhanced
Fatigue
Fear (specify focus)

Used with permission from NANDA International (2007). NANDA-I Nursing Diagnoses: Definitions and Classification 2007–2008. Philadelphia: NANDA-I.

Fluid Balance, readiness for enhanced
[Fluid Volume, deficient hyper/
  hypotonic]
Fluid Volume, deficient [isotonic]
Fluid Volume, excess
Fluid Volume, risk for deficient
Fluid Volume risk for imbalanced
Gas Exchange, impaired
Glucose, risk for unstable level
Grieving
Grieving, complicated
Grieving, risk for complicated
Growth, risk for disproportionate
Growth & Development, delayed
Health Behavior, risk prone
Health Maintenance, ineffective
Health-Seeking Behaviors (specify)
Home Maintenance, impaired
Hope, readiness for enhanced
Hopelessness
Human Dignity, risk for compromised
Hyperthermia
Hypothermia
Identify, disturbed personal
Immunization Status, readiness for enhanced
Infant Behavior, disorganized
Infant Behavior, organized, readiness for
  enhanced
Infant Behavior, risk for disorganized
Infant Feeding Pattern, ineffective
Infection, risk for
Injury, risk for
Injury, risk for perioperative positioning
Insomnia
Intracranial Adaptive Capacity, decreased
Knowledge, deficient [Learning Need] [specify]
Knowledge [specify], readiness for enhanced
Lifestyle, sedentary
Liver Function, risk for impaired
Loneliness, risk for
Memory, impaired
Mobility, impaired bed
Mobility, impaired physical
Mobility, impaired wheelchair
Moral Distress
Nausea
Noncompliance, [Adherence, ineffective]
  [specify]

Nutrition, less than body requirements,
  imbalanced
Nutrition, more than body requirements,
  imbalanced
Nutrition, readiness for enhanced
Nutrition, more than body requirements, risk
  for imbalanced
Oral Mucous Membrane, impaired
Pain, acute
Pain, chronic
Parenting, impaired
Parenting, readiness for enhanced
Parenting, risk for impaired
Perioperative Positioning, risk for
Peripheral Neurovascular Dysfunction, risk for
Poisoning, risk for
Post-Trauma Syndrome [specify stage]
Post-Trauma Syndrome, risk for
Power, readiness for enhanced
Powerlessness [specify level]
Powerlessness, risk for
Protection, ineffective
Rape-Trauma Syndrome
Rape-Trauma Syndrome: compound reaction
Rape-Trauma Syndrome: silent reaction
Religiosity, impaired
Religiosity, risk for impaired
Religiosity, readiness for enhanced
Relocation Stress Syndrome
Relocation Stress Syndrome, risk for
Role Performance, ineffective
Self-Care Deficit: bathing/hygiene
Self-Care Deficit: dressing/grooming
Self-Care Deficit: feeding
Self-Care Deficit: toileting
Self-Care, readiness for enhanced
Self-Concept, readiness for enhanced
Self-Esteem, chronic low
Self Esteem, situational low
Self Esteem, risk for situational low
Self-Mutilation
Self-Mutilation, risk for
Sensory Perception, disturbed: (specify:
  visual, auditory, kinesthetic, gustatory,
  tactile, olfactory)
Sexual Dysfunction
Sexuality Pattern, ineffective
Skin Integrity, impaired

Skin Integrity, risk for impaired
Sleep, readiness for enhanced
Sleep Deprivation
Social Interaction, impaired
Social Isolation
Sorrow, chronic
Spiritual Distress
Spiritual Distress, risk for
Spiritual Well-Being, readiness for enhanced
Stress Overload
Suffocation, risk for
Suicide, risk for
Surgical Recovery, delayed
Swallowing, impaired
Therapeutic Regimen Management, effective
Therapeutic Regimen Management, ineffective
Therapeutic Regimen Management, ineffective community
Therapeutic Regimen Management, ineffective family
Therapeutic Regimen Management, readiness for enhanced
Thermoregulation, ineffective
Thought Processes, disturbed

Tissue Integrity, impaired
Tissue Perfusion, ineffective (specify type: cerebral, cardiopulmonary, renal, gastrointestinal, peripheral)
Transfer Ability, impaired
Trauma, risk for
Unilateral Neglect Syndrome
Urinary Elimination, impaired
Urinary Elimination, readiness for enhanced
Urinary Incontinence, functional
Urinary Incontinence, overflow
Urinary Incontinence, reflex
Urinary Incontinence, stress
Urinary Incontinence, total
Urinary Incontinence, urge
Urinary Incontinence, risk for urge
Urinary Retention [acute/chronic]
Ventilation, impaired spontaneous
Ventilatory Weaning Response, dysfunctional
Violence, [actual/] risk for other-directed
Violence, [actual/] risk for self-directed
Walking, impaired
Wandering [specify sporadic or continual]
[ ] author recommendations

INDEX